G.L.O.W. Rx

YOUR PRACTICAL GUIDE TO RELEASING YOUR INHIBITIONS, FINDING YOUR PURPOSE, AND LIVING FREE, HEALTHY, & WHOLE

DR. NICOLE McCARTY

ISBN: (978-1-7359845-0-6)

Printed in the United States of America

DEDICATION

For Ember-Joi
There will never be anything you can't do! Here's to breaking
barriers and soaring as only eagles do. May God's grace take you
places your inheritance can't. You are my Why. Mommie loves you.

For Alani
You can be anything you desire! Love comes in many forms,
I'm so blessed my bonus was you. May you keep God first and
allow Him to direct your path. Mrs. Nicole loves you.

For Kamal
For the times when you pushed me to soar when I had only
the energy to fly. You are my heart. You are my love. With
God, we can do ANYTHING! Thank you, and I love you.

For Mommie, Grann & Papa
For every support and sacrifice you made to make sure I KNEW
I could DO and BE Anything. For embracing my unique
nature and free-spirited soul to help me to be the woman,
wife, and mother I am today...I love you, and I thank you.

WELLNESS CHEST

A GIFT FOR YOU...

As you prepare to start your journey to being healthy, whole, and happy, it was really important to me that you have a place to continue learning and growing in what is best for you. This is a place I can update on demand to serve you better, and the icing on the cake is it is **FREE**! This virtual platform essentially will become your Wellness Chest in which you can learn additional information about overall health, wellness, nutrition, fitness, stress management, and many other health-related concepts. You can access your Wellness Chest by visiting **www.drnicolemccarty.com/GLOWRx-WellnessChest**.

Inside the Wellness Chest is a treasure trove of health goodies for the mind, body, soul, and spirit. There is bonus content and a community of individuals on a similar health journey with whom you can GLOW and Grow together. Therefore, go ahead and get your access now by going to **www.drnicolemccarty.com/GLOWRx-WellnessChest**. This is your time to dedicate yourself to creating your **#GLOWRx** plan so that you can live Free, Healthy, and Whole.

Oh! One more thing...I'd love for you to tag me on Instagram **@dr.nicolemccarty** and use the hashtag **#GLOWRxBook** while you're there. Who in the world can't benefit from additional health and wellness knowledge? Do you know anyone? I don't. Let's take this journey, shall we. All it takes is a first step, and this is it! I'll see you inside!

PROLOGUE

G.L.O.W. *Grow & Live Optimally Well* is a mantra of sorts. It's the premise behind why I am where I am and why I do what I do. I became a doctor so that I could help people. That's only the most generic and laziest response one could ever give to the age-old question, "What made you want to become a doctor?"

Perhaps, I should offer something a little more... robust in thought. As a child, I was very active in the community because I came from a long line of educators and community leaders. My mom was an educator and software engineer. Brains and Beauty! (I totally took after her!) My grandparents were active and community pioneers in EVERYTHING! My grandmother was one of the first black department chairs at our community college, which is now a state institution, and a pioneer in the field of cosmetology and black hair care. My grandfather was one of the first and only black people at the time to work at Cape Canaveral, Florida, for Florida Power and Light as an engineer. He was a black supervisor when it wasn't very popular to have a black man in that position overseeing the nuclear division for a large portion of the South Florida coast. Community was very important to them. My grandmother was seemingly in every community organization and on every advisory board that existed on the planet! My grandfather was on most scenes with her, and he was a part of the founding golf club that mentors and gives back to the community even now. We ate like southerners, but we were always mindful of health. My mom has this knack for soulful cooking with a nutritional twist, so I had the best of foods in taste and preparation. My grandfather had a garden, so when we wanted fresh fruit and vegetables, we often were able to go pick fruit off the tree or pick vegetables from the garden at any given time. Basically, I had good roots. My upbringing gave me the foundation to understand the importance and gift of good health.

Fast forward...with these tools and knowledge, it's no surprise that God led me down a path of health and wellness. My passion and life principles from a young age have centered around the concept that health is wealth. Therefore, I went on to complete my B.S. in Cardiopulmonary Science after deciding that pharmacy (though a great career and program) just didn't measure up to my wellness lifestyle. I'm a firm believer in never doing what I wouldn't advise or advocate for myself or my family. It just wasn't my thing (even after they called my mom to try to change my mind). I knew there was something different God had in store for me. My first career as a respiratory therapist took me into specialty units and allowed me to learn specialty skills (brain injury rehabilitation, critical care, trauma, neonatal critical care, etc.) This is where I gained my experience in the allopathic field of medicine. My experiences were often exhilarating and different. I learned a lot in terms of politics, humanity, discipline, and compassion. It served me well and served a purpose.

As life would have it, I detoured into the field of education after a traumatic car accident derailed me from the allopathic model (traditional medical model of surgeries and pharmaceuticals) of health care. I went on to teach and coach an amazing group of students and student athletes in track and field and girls' weightlifting. This opportunity introduced me to chiropractic where I met a fellow believer and doctor who prophesied to me that I would be relocating to pursue my doctorate that following year. I laughed. Ha! The joke was on me. I believe Woody Allen coined the phrase, "If you really want to make God laugh, tell Him your plans." Well, He must have been cracking up that day because I just knew I wasn't relocating to start school for chiropractic. I was looking at Ph.D. programs in FL, or so I thought.

Welp! A year later, I started my doctorate in chiropractic, and life took off from there. I went on to complete my degree and started another degree program to complement it. After completing my M.S. in Sport Health Science with a concentration in Sport Injury Management, I practiced as a sports chiropractor and soft tissue specialist in both GA and SC. I also had the honor of teaching other master's and doctoral degree students in the subject areas of radiology, orthopedic diagnosis, physiotherapeutics, etc. Education has always been in my genes, I suppose, and now, I use those same skills to educate and coach my patients and clients.

Life was amazing, but it was life! I went through some growing pains personally at one point though. I endured a challenging relationship in which I lost who I was, what I wanted, and what I needed. I was just lost. The worst part was, I KNEW IT! I reached a point at which I had a pow wow with God about what I needed to do to exact change in my life because I knew I needed it. He told me that He needed me... just me. His words were, "Baby girl, I have everything you want in store for you, but I need you to let go of what you're holding onto and trust me." Well, I did, and just like that, I ended my engagement, relocated, and started over. Has God ever placed you in a situation in which you had to start over? I grew closer to God more than ever during this time. My intimacy increased, my discernment increased, and my ability to trust Him increased. My ability to love and appreciate myself increased, and I learned the art of letting go. It is an art...believe me.

Discernment is a learned skill, and I cultivated that bad boy. God also showed me who I was including the good, the bad, and the indifferent. I had to accept some ugly truths about myself so that I could change them and become the woman God designed me to be. Little did I know, God was setting me up for so much more. This was my rebirth, and I knew before I could walk into that place, I had to be comfortable, happy, and content with me. I remember having moments where I would cry but then I cried a little less. My tears became trophies that signified my growth. The growth in the internal makeup of who I was that no one could really see. There was no cheering section on social media, no fans, just me, Jesus, and a few close friends and family. As a result, when I did re-enter the dating market, I dated with purpose and found balance with potential realizing that there are no "ready-made" men but there are men and companions you can grow with and that's the beauty of the love God had for me. There is so much more to my testimony, but I'll stop there. Fast forward to now. I am married to an amazing and supportive man. I have a beautiful daughter, a bonus daughter, a wonderful family, and a loving village. I love my life and all of its imperfections, but most of all, I love this journey full of growth, freedom, healing, love, service, and abundance. All of my fundamentals resurfaced, and I can feel how my journey has prepared me for my purpose. It wasn't just about the physical health that made a difference. It was so much more than that. The mental, spiritual, and emotional aspects were just as important. From this rebirth came health and healing from the inside out. Even though I'd always owned who I was, this period of my life was when I took ownership. This time of birthing anew was when total and complete health and wellness became mine. It was much more than just the common buzz words of health and wealth because it was what the words represented. I was focused on health that *leads to* wealth in the quality of life that I was able to live. Being able to model what I preached and lived unapologetically in my truth gave me the freedom to build what I wanted other women to live just as I lived it, EACH AND EVERY DAY.

Hi! I am Dr. Nicole McCarty, and I am a life enthusiast! I love life and the blessings that come from it. Sure, I frown like anyone else when things are let's say…"less than optimal," but the biggest difference in my approach to life is that I don't stay in "frown town." Let's be honest, life absolutely can suck sometimes, BUT as bad as it may seem, it can turn around and make you absolutely beam from ear to ear. That's the beauty and versatility of life. My amazing bonus dad always would say, "Just wait a while. Things will change." Things never remain constant, but they *are* ever changing. It's up to us to choose the direction in which we move as they change. I made a promise a while ago after falling in love with myself again that I would never, ever, ever allow myself to get to that place again. The lessons I learned made me make fewer excuses than I ever have, and the direction I'm traveling makes me grow stronger so that I can have the sustainability to climb higher, run faster, dream bigger, and achieve heights previously unknown to me with clarity, patience (work in progress), and wisdom. I now G.L.O.W. unapologetically. It's your turn to do the same. It's amazing where I live. Won't you join me?

TABLE OF CONTENTS

PART 3: PHYSICALLY: HEALTH FROM THE INSIDE OUT

PART 4: EMOTIONALLY: MAKE TIME TO P.L.A.Y.

INTRODUCTION

I t's a familiar scene from one of my favorite movies. She's a woman who finds herself lost in who she is and what she wants, so she decides to leave it all to travel across the world on a journey of self-discovery after a failed marriage and some self-realization. In this scene, she's having what some might call a pity party as she talks about missing her ex-husband to her friend. What her friend says is pivotal in that moment. His response, "So miss him! Send him some light and love every time you think of him and drop him. You know, if you could clear out all that space in your mind that you're using to obsess over this guy and your failed marriage, you'd have a vacuum in a doorway. And do you know what the universe would do with that doorway? Whhhssshhh! It would rush in and fill you with more love than you've ever dreamed of. Groceries (this was his nickname for her), I think you have the capacity one day to love the whole world." The best part... the most integral part is when she asks, "When is the period of grieving going to pass?" His response, "You want a date on the calendar? NO, you've got to DO the Work!"

What does the "work" look like for you? Well, it's different for everyone, but everyone's work falls under the four pillars of health: health in your spirit, mind, body, and soul. Maybe you're not grieving a relationship or a person, but perhaps, it's a situation or circumstances. Perhaps, it's YOU. You may be grieving the person you once were or one you thought you wanted to be. There is no harm in missing people and things. We are human. What we need to hear sounds much like the counsel he gave his friend in the movie which is to miss whatever it may be for you, send whatever that is some light, and love and drop it. Move forward and allow the love of the healthiest version of yourself to rush in so that you have the capacity to love others *adequately*.

YES, this book is about health but not the surface definition of abs and buns. It's about the legacy you want to leave for yourself, your children, your family, and your community. It's about the impact you want to have on those with whom you share time and space. It is about the love you want to have for yourself and others. The crazy thing about health is that it doesn't come to you via osmosis. It comes from educating yourself, understanding your needs, making the commitment, and taking the leap forward into it to walk it out day by day. What's crazier is that it's not a perfect science. It's a journey uniquely tailored to you, and like any journey, there will be days when you are tired, and you choose to rest. There will be days when you will be tired, and you will continue to push. There will be days when you will make the most optimal choices, and there will be days when you make the less optimal ones. Guess what? ALL of THIS is a part of the journey, your journey. Though your journey may share some similarities with others. Please understand, however, that your journey is still yours to take.

What good is a journey without a guide? Is it still effective? Of course it is, but a guide is a person or structure that shows you the way to others or directs your motion or positioning. Not only that, the guide oftentimes sees things and helps you circumvent pitfalls which saves you time and effort. (Insert why you've chosen G.L.O.W.) This book and its accompanying *G.L.O.W. Rx Transformation Guide* will help you build or rebuild a healthy lifestyle for you and those you love. What makes a guide so vital for change is that it's built on the constructs of a solid foundation. The foundational pillars of health are spiritual health, mental health, physical health, and emotional health. These four pillars create support for the monument that is You. As you journey through each section, we will unpack, provide clarity and instruction on spiritual health, and share how it relates to the mind body connection.

You'll even grab a few anatomy lessons along the way. It's your body, and you're in it EVERY MINUTE OF EVERY DAY. Why wouldn't you want to learn a little more about how your temple functions? This is not only meant to be informative, but also it is designed for true application. After all, you can have all of the knowledge in the world, but if you don't apply it, it is of little benefit to you. Lack of application, on the other hand, can be detrimental, so I wrote this book to take the guesswork out of it. I wanted to give you enough information so that you understand WHY you are doing something as opposed to doing it simply because I said so.

Your journey will begin with exploring the mind-body connection along with tools and exercises to apply what you learn. We are doing more than just reading here. Have you ever tried meditation? It's powerful, and guess what, God honors it. (I practice meditation from a Christian perspective. Yes, it's a thing, and it's awesome!) Don't just take my word for it. Dive in, and you just might surprise yourself with what you learn and how that changes your life. Remember those anatomy lessons I just mentioned? Well, it's important to know that structure dictates function, and function dictates application. Exploring the mind-body connection is how you link your physical body to your spiritual roots and create a foundation for prayer or spiritual communication no matter which form you choose. **This is how we PRAY.**

Your journey continues in the next section as we address the mind to build mental health. Stress can be deadly. That's not a scare tactic. It is a fact. However, what is vital to your ability to enjoy your quality of life is how you manage the stressors in your life. I'm a firm believer that you can't change what you can't see. As you journey and journal through the chapters and exercises, you'll learn how to define, identify, prioritize, manage, and conquer your stresses. This process incorporates a number of perspective shifts and physical practices. Whenever you are stressed, one of the primary physical effects is the breath. Think of the last time you were under immense stress. How did it make you feel? I highly doubt it made you feel warm and fuzzy. I'm guessing that you may have experienced any number of things which included a headache, tightness in the neck and shoulders, elevated breath rate and heart rate, etc. Sound familiar? So, in this section, we conquer through our breath. **This is how we BREATHE.**

As you continue on, you will venture into the pillar of physical health. In this section, you'll learn about the standard definition of health. Here, you'll explore how you eat, sleep, and move since ALL are essential to life. Don't allow anyone to tell you otherwise. This is where you tackle different forms of nutrition and various theories on how to consume what is best for you based on who you are. More than just food, we have to "move it, move it," and let's be honest, sometimes, routines can get stale, and boredom can set in with the monotony of doing the same thing over and over and over again. Why not switch it up? Then, eventually, your body will need rest. Adequate rest is non-negotiable, or at least it should be, and you'll learn why. It just might change your mind about constantly pulling those popular all-nighters. There is magic that happens inside of our body when we sleep, so don't be that guy who kills the magic show. **This is how we EAT.**

As the journey comes to a pause because the journey only ends when you do, you are reintroduced to who you are in all of your unprecedented beauty. Here, you are reminded of your importance, your vitalism, and your worth. In this section, you re-learn how to ask and command from others what you require. To G.L.O.W. is to *Grow & Live Optimally Well.* As you retain your GLOW and shine brighter, you instinctively inspire others to do the same. It's not about living a perfect life; it's about being healthy and whole. To live whole is to live complete in yourself. It doesn't mean that you have to be perfect by any means. We aren't perfect, and life won't be either, but it does mean that you will commit to live your entire life in a state of being whole, unbroken, and undamaged. The moments you will experience inevitably may be heartbreaking and damaging, but the G.L.O.W. that exudes from within you will come from a WHOLE place, a WELL place. **This is how we LOVE.**

Allow me to share with you my inspiration for this manual of sorts. The scene above is from one of my favorite movies, *EAT, PRAY, LOVE* starring Julia Roberts (who is an amazing actress by the way). This movie is based on the book by Elizabeth Gilbert. The story line focuses on a woman who by most traditional standards had everything (marriage, successful career, house, etc.) only to find that she was empty, lost, and unhappy. She decides to take the leap and find herself again after a chance encounter with an oracle. She embarks on a journey of self-discovery and healing that leads her to delight in eating in Italy, experience prayer in India, and find balance, inner peace, and inadvertently true love in Bali. Now, I'm not saying that you will find the man or woman of your dreams at the end of this book, but I will say that if you commit to yourself and the process, YOUR process, then you will find the YOU of your dreams as you EAT, PRAY, BREATHE and LOVE yourself to a Well YOU and a Whole YOU.

PART 1

SPIRITUALLY: THE MIND-BODY CONNECTION

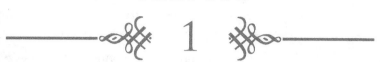

1

WHAT IS THE MIND-BODY CONNECTION?

I was speaking with a friend the other day, and she pondered the question of purpose. She expressed the following feelings and emotions. "I've studied the field of computer science for 17 years with 10 years of experience at least, and I'm just not happy, but I don't know why I'm not happy. On top of that, I just feel like I'm existing. I'm tired, moody, and maybe even borderline depressed. I'm just here, and I don't know how to move from here because I don't know my purpose, and I don't know how to find my purpose."

Hmmm…Have you ever been here because I have? There is nothing worse than feeling like you simply are going through the motions day in and day out with no progress, no happiness, and no feeling of fulfillment to accompany it. Purpose is one of those funny things though. It is the ultimate unicorn of life. Yes, I said unicorn. You know, it's the elusive mythical creature that is impossible to catch except for the fact that you actually can catch it, tap into it, ignite it, embrace it, share it, serve it, and GLOW from it. Ha! See what I did there?

To find your purpose and tap into it, you first have to know and fully understand what it is you are searching to find. Therefore, let's perform a brief dissection to aid you along your journey. Purpose has many meanings in many cultures, but what does this mean for you? When you lead a purpose-driven life, you thrive where you are. What you do empowers you to keep going, and you feel fulfilled, right? The one thing that prevents many people from finding their purpose is having an established mind-body connection. It seems unrelated, doesn't it, but follow me. This connection connects the energy and functionality of your body with that of your mind to complete a very clear circle and path towards determining your God-ordained passion and purpose. Think of it as "clearing the clutter." How does purpose exist in a disconnected and disjointed space?

In order to explore the mind-body connection, you first must establish and know what it is. For centuries, healers have pondered the connection between mental and physical health. Yet, in recent years, science finally has begun to recognize and acknowledge the powerful connections through which emotional, spiritual, and behavioral factors can affect health outcomes directly (Weinberg, 2017). This discovery is not new by any means. Our ancestors and virtually every system of medicine in the world dating back 300 years treated the mind and body as a whole. During the 17th century, the Western world started to view the mind and body as two distinct entities. In this approach, they viewed the body like a machine that was complete with independent and replaceable parts with no connection whatsoever to the mind. Don't get me wrong, I'm not saying this was all bad. In fact, this laid the groundwork for many of the advances we have in medicine, surgery, trauma care, pharmaceuticals, and various other aspects of allopathic medicine. For example, surgeries, pharmaceuticals, etc. allow treatment of independent body parts and ailments. However, these very advances left us with a void in the importance and significance of that same scientific inquiry into human beings' emotional and spiritual lives and their resounding impact on healing and lifestyle. However, as our culture changes, we not only see the integration of the mind-body connection back into the allopathic model of health, but also we witness the surging growth of other healthcare disciplines that focus more on integrative health therapies and the mind-body connection like chiropractic medicine, naturopathic medicine, Chinese medicine, etc.

As we conduct more research into the mind-body concept, we are finding that emotions and thought patterns can contribute to imbalances within the body. The beliefs you hold about yourself and the world, along with your emotions, your memories, and your habits can influence your mental and physical health. These connections between what is going on in your mind and heart and what is happening in your body form the psycho-emotional roots of health and disease. Do you remember singing "Dem Bones" as a kid? Let me help jog your memory. "The leg bone is connected to the knee bone. The knee bone is connected to the thigh bone. The thigh bone is connected to the hip bone. Now, shake them skeletal bones." The key point here is that all of your bones are connected. Well, guess what? EVERYTHING in your body that makes up who you are both inside and outside is CONNECTED. One of the most important and most forgotten connections is that of the mind and body. This connection, I would argue, is vital for a successful and effective existence. Let's take a closer look at the mind-body connection and its role in health and wellness.

The mind-body connection experiences various mental states that are collectively labeled the "mind." While most people consider the mind to be synonymous with the brain, they are two separate and distinct entities. How you think, how you feel, and what you believe are characteristic states of your "mind". Let's use technology to demonstrate this example. Since technology is all around us, let's look at the widely used computer for instance. In order for your computer to run and perform all of the many tasks you ask, or shall I say command of it, it requires software in the form of programs, operating systems, and applications. You can say the brain is analogous to the hardware of a computer, and the mind is analogous to the software on the computer. Without the software, the computer hardware becomes a glorified and moderately costly paperweight.

When I worked as a respiratory therapist, I had the opportunity to work in a brain injury rehabilitation unit. I particularly loved my days when I had rounds with patients in this unit because they were sweet and without inhibitions. I remember a few occasions when we had therapy students shadow us during our shifts. One day, I had a student who needed an additional explanation about what made this unit so unique and why the behavior of the patients was so incredibly diverse and different from one room to the next. I recall explaining that a patient who made a few advances was impaired due to his brain injury. I explained to the student that although it was not apparent to people when they first met the patient that there was something wrong, once they began conversing with the patient, it was obvious that there was a bit of a disconnect that caused the patient to have altered or impaired behaviour. The injury was in the brain although the patient's mind was intact. Similarly, while I was a student studying to be a respiratory therapist, I had rotations through a psychiatric facility. In this instance, there were patients who had an impairment in their minds and not in their brains. An example of this was a patient on one of my rotations at the time who was brilliant. He had writings and formulas plastered everywhere and had multiple doctorates. His history however, was that of a psychotic break. His brain was still very much functional and brilliant, but his approach to life had become chaotic and disillusioned. The mind and the brain are connected but two separate entities intertwined with each other.

As a part of this hardware to software connection, there are also very important and necessary supporting characters. Chemical messengers like hormones and neurotransmitters allow constant communication between the mind and various systems of the body that include the nervous, endocrine, immune, cardiovascular, digestive, and musculoskeletal systems. Neurological pathways act as exits and roads that feed into a major interstate by connecting parts of the brain that process emotions with the spinal cord, muscles, cardiovascular system, and digestive tract. These pathways allow major life events, stressors, or emotions to trigger physical symptoms in each of the systems connected to the brain, which is ALL of them, and cause some systems to be affected more than others. In this analogy, think of your life events and stressors like car accidents that happen on the interstate. Have you ever been in traffic for hours and had to take detours to side streets and back roads to get to your destination only to find that those side streets were also congested because everyone had the same idea? Well, the same thing happens in your body. That "collision of emotions and life" occurs, and whether it's good or bad, you can experience physical symptoms that are indicative of the mind-body connection. Your mind and its mental states connect to your body and send it signals that something is affecting you adversely. Some examples include the butterfly or queasy feeling in your stomach when you are nervous, the feeling that your heart is going to pound out of your chest when you are angry, stressed or nervous, and the tightness in your muscles when you are chronically stressed or responding to a stressful event.

Similar to the roadway analogy, these systems intersect to establish the mind-body connection that influences your health. This connection is so powerful, unbreakable, and influential, that it is a major determining factor in how you are able to maintain your health for optimal living or how you allow it to degrade, which leads to the development of disease. Which trajectory you choose is paramount to life. Negative emotions like fear, anxiety, or anger activate the part of the brain known as the amygdala. This activation increases the production of stress hormones, which may suppress the immune system and set the stage for the development of infections or cancer by slowing the body's ability to recover from stresses and trauma. Have you ever been in a place where you were just stressed? I remember a time in my life when I was going through it! I had recently ended an engagement. I was traveling out of state on a weekly basis, working two to three jobs, and trying to throw my hat in the ring in the over-35 dating pool. It was crazy, and all of that stress culminated in my resistance becoming lowered and leaving me vulnerable to the flu. It was pretty bad. Come to think of it, all of the times I've come down with the flu occurred when my stress levels were through the roof. Each time, the flu knocked me out, and it took me about two weeks to fully recover. Stress will keep you strangled, struggling, gasping for air, and unable to recover. I seriously had to learn to let some things go to create a space where my body could heal and become whole.

On the other hand, positive emotions trigger "reward" pathways located deep in the area of the brain known as the ventral striatum. Positive emotions create a lasting activation that leads to greater feelings of well-being. The more positive you feel about yourself and your environment around you, the lower your stress and the hormones associated with it will be. These lower levels in stress hormones yield resilience. Resilience in the "emotionally well" doesn't mean that you don't experience difficulties, but rather, it means that you are able to bounce back from difficulties faster. You are better able to avoid dwelling on negative thoughts and appreciate the good times. Additionally, developing a sense of meaning and purpose in life contributes to a healthy state of being emotionally well which allows you to focus on what's most important to you. For instance, have you ever awakened on the RIGHT side of the bed? Man! On those mornings, I'm feeling good. I'm looking good, and I'm feeling like nothing or no one can stop me. Most times, when I own those feelings, my day is pretty seamless. I can accomplish more. I feel beautiful. The sun is shining, and the birds are singing. I even find myself with a little pep in my step, and in the words of Ice Cube, "Today was a good day." Don't you want to have a good day? We should have them every day if I'm being completely honest. Think of it this way, you get to look good and serve out of your abundance while giving to others out of the surplus you have within you. #Winning

Now that you know that biological functioning can be affected positively or negatively by different mental states, it is important for you to know that there are vibrations that correspond with those thoughts and emotions that occur in the mind and body. Yes, I said vibrations.

Vibrations are exactly what you think they are - very fast, oscillating movements in the body. The body is always vibrating....ALWAYS. Scientists have determined that some of our most basic and vital physiological processes generate mechanical vibrations at very low frequencies to produce the heartbeat, respirations, circulation or blood flow, etc. To put it in context, one of my patients asked me one day, "So Doc, you mean to tell me that my cells are vibrating right now? Like, right now? Like, my cell phone?" I chuckled a bit, but my answer was "YES! Exactly like your cell phone." Our thoughts and emotions carry vibrations that greatly impact our overall physiological state even down to the cellular and biochemical level. On the physical level alone, the body is made up of cells, atoms, and water in a constant state of motion which creates energy that dictates and influences structure and function. To put it into perspective, scientists estimate that there are almost 200 trillion atoms in just 1 cell and roughly 100 trillion cells in the average human body!! This yields a 2 with 24-26 zeros after it! That's A LOT of vibrating!

With that vibrating, science also demonstrates that thoughts, words, and feelings have the ability to change the structure and function of cells, atoms, and water in the body. This concept sheds new light on the childhood phrase, "Sticks and stones may break my bones, but words will never hurt me." Words are powerful. The Bible even confirms this in Proverbs 18:21. It says, "Death and life are in the power of the tongue, and those who love it will eat its fruit." Positive, kind, and inspiring thoughts and emotions vibrate in harmony with your cells since they share a similar frequency that allows them to function optimally. If positive words vibrate in harmony with our cells, then it's safe to say that negative words do not.

When we apply those conflicting vibrations of our cells and atoms that make up our genetic code, the unstable proteins created from those discordant materials end up becoming the building blocks of the body. It's like the childhood story, "The Three Little Pigs." Would you rather have your house built of bricks or straw? This importance encourages you to choose and use your words wisely. This reality gives credence to the rationale that supports the effectiveness of techniques like affirmations and hypnotherapy on both the body and the mind. The famous philosopher, Descartes, said, "I think therefore I am." The Bible says, "As a man thinketh in his heart, so is he." (Proverbs 23:7) The natural pattern that exists is your thoughts become words, and your words become actions. Therefore, when you factor in the associated vibratory components that compound the health of your mind and body, the result becomes habits and behaviours that are put into practice on a consistent basis. Subsequently, your health is dependent upon the condition of repetitious thoughts, words, actions, and behaviors.

Now that we have a better understanding of what the mind-body connection is, we can begin to explore purpose and the process that people use to find it. The largest hindrance in establishing that mind-body connection is knowing yourself. You can't begin to find your purpose or know what it is without first taking a good look at who you are from the inside out and being OK with the fact that this will most likely and most certainly change as you develop, grow, and reach new heights. Second to knowing yourself is liking yourself. This is discussed in more detail later in the book; however, explore the basics of getting to know and like yourself so that you can learn to love yourself and others effectively. This self-love is one of the key components to living your best life and becoming a healthier you.

In my research, I've found a wonderful narrative that demonstrates the pathway connecting purpose to self-exploration. Farnoosh Brock writes, "At the core of our desires is living a life of purpose and meaning. At the core of a life of purpose and meaning is being of service to others. At the core of being of service to others is finding peace and happiness. At the core of finding peace and happiness, we discover Who We Are." What good is living this beautiful life if we don't live it with authenticity and pride. Everything we do for ourselves and others is predicated on who we are intertwined with what our purpose is. When we know this, we can experience true happiness outside of circumstances.

The irony in "knowing" yourself is perhaps the fact that you are probably the person you know the least. You've only spent your whole existence together, yet you lack the intimacy and relationship required to cultivate a healthy connection that makes you whole. Please understand that this is not about a personality test or knowing your favorite color or favorite food. Those factors are most certainly complementary. This version of knowing yourself is much greater, and the stakes are higher. The consequences of *not* knowing who you are can prove to be more costly and detrimental to you and those attached to you. You are essentially talking about who you are at your core when no one is watching. Knowing what matters most to you is what makes you come alive. It is also what feeds your soul and drains your spirit. Once you get to know yourself, the next step is taking that knowledge and using it to understand WHY you are WHERE you are and establishing HOW to make the best choices for you. This powerful transformation will propel you forward in life and give you the courage to take a stand, take a leap, and soar to your destiny.

Be mindful that this is an introspective journey and a personal one. It's easy to look at others and assume they've mastered the art of knowing themselves. I have a few rules, but this leads me to one...well, two of them. Number #1: Don't ever make assumptions; Number #2: Don't be fooled by what you see because there is often more to it than meets the eye. When it comes to purpose, people tend to approach it one of two ways. They either treat purpose like this elusive unicorn or mythical creature that is impossible to catch, or they treat it like it's the gift that keeps on giving, meaning that the initial gift is the blessing, and the service to others is continual. What differentiates these two rules is the alignment component. To be aligned simply means to be in order. Is your purpose intentional and in order as it serves both you and those around you?

Many wonder if it's possible to live a life that demonstrates purposeful alignment. I assure you, it is. I'm living proof. Perhaps the better question is, is there a difference in being aligned with your purpose and walking in your purpose? The answer to that is yes. When you know yourself, not only are you better able to recognize opportunities that align with your purpose, but also once you are aligned, you can flow, walk, run, and fly in your purpose by knowing what to choose and what to decline. The difference is in the prepositions "in" and "with." Merriam Webster defines the word "with" as a function word that indicates a participant in an action, transaction, or arrangement. While "in" is defined as a function word that indicates inclusion, location, or position within limits, or it is used as a function word that indicates purpose. To be aligned *with* your purpose means your actions are congruent with your purposed desire. When you walk *in* your purpose, you essentially embody that purposed desire and become one with it. There are a lot of people who don't know themselves, but the great thing is that YOU don't have to be one of them. If you're asking yourself, "How do I get to know myself really well?" One simple way to do that is to learn your values, passions, and goals. In order to evaluate these things, it's simply a matter of asking the right questions. It takes time, so you must remember to be patient with yourself. It's only your life's work on the line.

So, now it's action time. You'll need your G.L.O.W. Rx Transformation Guide for this one. Refer to Experience 1.1 These questions are important to ask because they prompt the process of self-inquiry. Like working out, the hardest part is getting started. As you begin, it may seem unfamiliar, but as the process unfolds, the questions become easier and maybe even a little fun. Sometimes, you might find that either you don't know, or you are afraid to believe how awesome you really are. My advice to you is simply take the good, the bad, and the indifferent. One of my favorite quotes (and there are a number of them) is by Marianne Williamson. It comes from her New York Times bestseller and first book, *A Return to Love: Reflections on the Principles of "A Course in Miracles"*. This quote became my personal mantra of sorts. It reminds me of the awesomeness inside of me and inspires me to share and spread the message to others.

Our deepest fear is not that we are inadequate. Our deepest fear is that we are powerful beyond measure. It is our light, not our darkness that most frightens us. We ask ourselves, ' who am I to be brilliant, gorgeous, talented, fabulous?' Actually, who are you not to be? You are a child of God. Your playing small does not serve the world. There is nothing enlightened about shrinking so that other people won't feel insecure around you. We are all meant to shine, as children do. We were born to make manifest the glory of God that is within us. It's not just in some of us; it's in everyone. And as we let our own light shine, we unconsciously give other people permission to do the same. As we are liberated from our own fear, our presence automatically liberates others. (Williamson, 2014)

My GLOW Up

We have had a connection with our cells since our conception, and this connection increased in its tangibility when we were born. Most of us, as we get older and mature, ignore this powerful connection and become so inundated with socialization that we forget to socialize with ourselves. For instance, when was the last time you took yourself out on a date by yourself to the movies, your favorite restaurant, or the spa? When was the last time that it was just you in all your splendor and no one else to accompany you? Socializing with yourself helps you remain connected with who you are, what you like, and what you enjoy when no one else is around. Socializing with yourself removes your dependence on others to make you whole. Losing that connection with ourselves blocks us from understanding our God-given purpose because we are missing the critical piece of knowing ourselves enough to be purposeful. Reestablishing that connection subsequently can reconnect us to our journey, vision, purpose, and most importantly, ourselves.

CHAPTER

2

MEDITATION...WHAT IS IT? HOW DO I DO...IT?

I was sitting in a room filled with about 9 ladies that I'd known for maybe 6 months, and suddenly, my yoga instructor said that we were going to meditate. My initial thought was, "Meditate? Who has time to sit still for 15 minutes and do nothing without sneaking in a nap?" Now, I'd been in yoga classes and *attempted* to meditate previously, and well, let's just say that it was really easy for me to "blend in." When I studied for my yoga teacher certification, I knew I had to learn how to meditate, yet it seemed intimidating and daunting to me. After all, I am a free spirit who, like a diamond, has many facets. My mind never shuts off, and if I'm honest, it still doesn't except when I'm meditating. I'm always a work in progress. Here I was, preparing to assume my meditative posture with the idea being that I would sit still with a focused mind for 15 minutes. It seemed like a preposterous thought, but I did it...sort of! I worked my way through it one step at a time. Here I was, nowhere to run or hide, and I was about to embark upon a journey that would soon change my life. I'm still on that journey even now; however, I'm loving every minute of it.

When most people think of the word, "meditation," what comes to their minds is peace, but the visual usually consists of individuals seated in a quiet space in relaxed clothing with their eyes closed, and nothing is happening around them. (Think about a monk in a monastery). This visualization evokes a spirit of peace if one imagined himself or herself there. However, meditation is so much more than that. The goal is to accompany meditation *with* mindfulness (yes, those are different) and enter a place of awareness where most of us have never ventured. Sounds super deep, right? Yeah, well, it is...sort of.

The two terms: *meditation* and *mindfulness* are often used synonymously when in actuality, they are distinctly different. Meditation is a way to train the mind. Think of the mind like any muscle in the body. It takes training and conditioning to get it into tip top shape. It's not just a one-time instance either. It is something that requires consistent training for optimal operation and function. The same rules apply with the mind.

Merriam-Webster defines *meditation* or the root word, *meditate,* as "the ability to engage in contemplation or reflection or to engage in mental exercise such as concentration on one's breathing or repetition of a mantra for the purpose of reaching a heightened level of spiritual awareness." *Mindfulness*, on the other hand, is defined as "the practice of maintaining a non-judgmental state of heightened or complete awareness of one's thoughts, emotions, or experiences on a moment to moment basis." Put more simply, meditation is the training of the mind or better yet the training of our attention.

Most of the time, our minds are wandering. We are either thinking about the future, dwelling on the past, worrying, fantasizing, fretting, stressing, daydreaming, or any combination of those mental actions. Not only does meditation bring you back to the present moment and bring that moment into focus, but also it gives you clarity, more importantly, to use tools to manage your stresses effectively so that you exist in much calmer and kinder spaces. This process benefits you and those around you. By training your attention or your ability to focus or be attentive, you gain the ability to step out of those distracting thoughts and allow yourself to arrive in the present moment with clarity and balance. Mindfulness, on the other hand, is simply the experience of (the mind) being present and aware in the moment without reflexive judgement, automatic criticism, or mind wandering. Through a concerted and very intentional effort, we are able to incorporate that practice throughout the day. Creating this positive habit and strategy allows us to activate it during the most difficult times.

Contrary to popular belief, the goal of mindfulness is neither to stop thinking nor to empty the mind. I don't even think that is possible. Instead, the goal is all about control. Oftentimes, it's comfortable to allow emotions, thoughts, and beliefs to consume and dictate your actions and reactions to life's circumstances. Mindfulness encourages you to pay close attention to your physical sensations, thoughts, and emotions so that you may see them more clearly. With clear sight, we are able to assess and understand without making so many assumptions or making up stories. So, let's try it. The simplicity of this process is deceiving, but I'd like you to just be here, present, and focused...in this moment... right now, where you are without daydreaming or wandering.

Go on...try it.

Close your eyes and take a deep breath first.

Like right now.

I'll wait.

Are you back? How did it go? It is not as easy as it sounds, right? We just don't realize how imaginative we are until we intentionally try not to be imaginative. Don't get me wrong, being imaginative isn't bad. In fact, it's the total opposite. It's what drives innovation, but with that success and accomplishment comes the need for mental rest. The practice of mindful meditation can yield profound results which give us greater control of our actions and make room for more kindness and balance despite what's happening around us. Now, tell me you don't need more of that in your life. The most valuable result of mindfulness meditation is equanimity, which helps us understand better what causes stress and what we can do to prevent, address, or relieve it.

Where some people get hung up is the derivation of mindfulness and meditation. There's a misconception that mindfulness is religious. It is not. The reality is that while this practice is popular in the Buddhist culture, the actions exist outside of any religion or culture. I practice mindfulness in my specialty of yoga from a Christian perspective. If anything, mindfulness is a simple technique for mental strengthening and stress reduction. There are no boundaries to it because it is self-care. There is no comparison because the journey is specific to each individual. Take this moment and ponder the answer to this question, "How often do you take time for yourself?" By taking time for yourself, I don't mean the type of self-care that is involved in getting your hair or nails done or even treating yourself to a spa treatment. What I mean by self-care is taking care of the innermost parts of you. These are the parts that no one sees and the parts that don't require action from anyone else but you. THAT is self-care. Now, I'll ask the question again. "How often do you engage in self-care?" For many, your second answer may be a little different than your original answer. If it is, that means you've got the concept! You know the difference! "Knowing is half the battle..." G.I. Joe anyone?

There are several different types of meditation, and the most popular ones are mindfulness meditation and transcendental meditation. Mindfulness meditation is the most common form, (which we've discussed above) and the latter is gaining more and more popularity because it aims to promote a state of relaxed awareness through the recitation of a mantra. The others include gazing, breath, imagery, and physical sensations. Let's briefly explore the five different focal points you can use when meditating.

It is important to know that the first stage of meditation is concentrating on a specific object or establishing a focal point with the eyes open or closed. The use of sound in meditation is known as either a mantra or chanting. Many people are uncomfortable with the idea of chanting, but we essentially do it every day in music. Music uses repetitive phrases, correct? A mantra employs the use of a particular sound, phrase, or affirmation as a point of focus. If we dissect the word "mantra," we find that "man" means "to think," and "-tra", suggests "instrumentality." Therefore, you can think of a mantra as an instrument of thought. Whether you are reciting a mantra, contemplative prayer, or an affirmation, you should state it with purpose, feeling, and intentionality. This isn't something you say just to utter words. Just like anything else, you get out of it what you put into it. Therefore, this requires conscious engagement during your practice.

An extension of the mantra is chanting which involves both rhythm and pitch. While using a mantra can be relatively easy for beginners to use in their meditation, chanting often may be a little more intimating. For example, one of my favorite mantras is the phrase, "more than enough." Please understand that it takes time. It took time for me, and in the spirit of full transparency, I still don't chant often in my meditation. I remember being exposed to chanting in my first yoga class years ago. I totally felt like I was cheating on God, and worse yet, I felt that I had been sucked into the twilight zone. I didn't understand it. It was new and uncomfortable. Fast forward to me sitting in my yoga teacher certification course and chanting as if I had been doing it for years. My teacher used this simple example that made it click. She said a song is simply a chant put over music. Aha! Just like that, it made sense! While I'm still a work in progress when it comes to that one, I understand it, and for me, that's all I need to give it my all. I do utilize mantras and often substitute or infuse scriptures as my mantra for a certain practice or worship sequence.

Another use of establishing a focal point that is often fairly easy for beginners is using imagery. Traditionally, a meditator visualizes his/her chosen deity in a vivid and detailed fashion. During my 200-hour yoga teacher training (Yoga from a Christian Perspective), my instructor, Dayna Gelinas, would have us visualize getting into an elevator and traveling infinitely to the top to sit with Christ Jesus. I'll walk you through a meditative practice that utilizes imagery in your Wellness Chest so make sure you check the link in the front of the book to gain access. As a believer whose foundation is rooted in Christ, using Him as the focal point in my imagery is comforting and eases the process of meditating. Other pieces of imagery often used by others include natural objects like a flower, the ocean, or chakras, which are the energy centers of the body. An additional variation of using imagery is to maintain an open-eyed focus upon an object. This focus is referred to as a drishti, which means to view or gaze. The choices available here are limitless, but a candle flame is popular due to its symbolism for illuminating the mind for clarity of vision and purpose.

One of my favorite techniques is using the breath as a point of focus. Meditating on the breath doesn't require counting or any specific focusing methods, it really means just purely observing the breath as it is without changing it in any way. When you do this, you observe every nuance of the breath and each sensation it produces: how it moves in your abdomen and torso, how it feels as it moves in and out of your nose, what is its quality, what is its temperature, what is its texture, etc. Though you fully are aware of all of these details, you don't dwell on them or judge them. You simply remain detached from what you're observing. You serve as only a spectator. Don't try to analyze the breath. It is neither good nor bad. It is yours for you to be present with it from one moment to the next. Because transcendental meditation uses the breath in it, people oftentimes establish breath as a point of their focus with mindfulness meditation. The key to successful meditation is to use the instrument that works best for you.

The last focal point that we can use in meditation is watching physical sensations which resemble breathing because your focus heightens your senses. If you've ever closed your eyes and taken a few deep breaths, you might notice that upon doing so, you can identify certain aspects or characteristics of the breath (texture, temperature, etc.) that you wouldn't normally notice in everyday breathing. By removing one of your senses, your mind is able to focus more intently on your breathing. It works the same way with physical sensations. In this context, you will look deeply at a particular sensation that draws your attention. For example, look at how hot or cold your hands feel or concentrate on a physical or emotional area of discomfort. You must remember that whatever you choose remains your focal point for the entire practice. Some find that observing a physical sensation is more challenging than observing breath. When you are beginning, it is easy to find yourself drifting into sensory overload with some of these options. I completely understand. Please know that it is a part of the process and the practice.

My suggestion would be to sample all of the different focal points and create a mental list for the ones you like. You may prefer more tangible ways to calm scattered thoughts like mantras, chants, and visualizations. Get to know a part of you rarely accessible and learn about your inner workings from the inside out with breath and physical sensations. It is possible that different situations or temperaments may require different focal points. Having your favorites is nice, but you never know when you may want or need to try something a little different, so you should incorporate them all into your practice regimen. When you are able to divert your focus to just be present in the moment, wonderful things happen mentally, spiritually, emotionally, and physically.

By now, you may be asking yourself, "If meditation does all of this good and helps with stress reduction so much, why don't more people do it?" Well, what's the number one reason people don't venture out to try something new, taste a new food, listen to a different genre of music, or try a new career path? One word...FEAR. Fear of the unknown is a real thing in our culture, and the unfortunate part is that when we are fearful, we tend to pass on these fearful perspectives and ideologies to our children. Do we really want them to grow up in a world where the expectation is for them to be comfortable with the status quo? Absolutely not! My prayer and my desire is for them to grow up with discipline and proportional determination to DO anything and BE anything they want to be without limitations and misconceptions.

Let's explore the most common misconceptions (excuses) related to meditation. The most popular reasons I've heard are:

1. "I don't have time, and I don't know how."
2. "I'm afraid to be alone with my thoughts."
3. "I'm not doing it right."
4. "My mind is too scattered. I won't get anything out of it."
5. "I don't have enough discipline to stick with it."

We'll talk about each one individually.

1. "I DON'T HAVE TIME, AND I DON'T KNOW HOW."

Let's be honest (I'm a straight shooter), we tend to make time for what we want. If we do not know how to do something, technology has blessed us and made it easy for us to learn how to do it. With a few keystrokes and button clicks, we can learn almost anything. Now that we've gotten that part out of the way, let's go into how we can make the adjustments necessary to change the excuse statement above.

Transformation doesn't happen in one fell swoop. It happens incrementally. Short stints of meditation can lead to lasting changes. When I say short stints, I mean as little as five minutes. Just five minutes a day can yield results that reduce stress and increase focus, so you should start by carving out time each day. To start, you have to cultivate your environment, so you should sit comfortably in a quiet space on the floor (cushions can increase the comfort) or in a chair with your spine erect. Be sure you aren't slumped, or your back is not overarched. You should be moderately comfortable and not strained. I say moderately comfortable because any time you place the body in a new position, you may feel a little discomfort or unfamiliarity. If necessary, lie down (though

I would advise against this if you are tired or sleepy), close your eyes, and take a few deep breaths.

As you inhale, feel the air enter your nostrils and move down and fill your chest and abdominal cavity as the air causes it to rise and fall. As you exhale, release the air and empty it out through your mouth. Then, let your attention rest on your natural rhythm of breathing. If your mind wanders, don't fret. Instead, take notice of what has captured your attention and instead of allowing those thoughts to take root, let go of those thoughts or feelings and return your awareness and attention back to your breath. If you practice like this for a dedicated period of time each day, you then create a habit (See, some habits are good for you). Creating this habit provides you the ability to use it as a tool in your arsenal that allows you to call on mindfulness in any situation and circumstance.

2. "I'M AFRAID TO BE ALONE WITH MY THOUGHTS, AND I DON'T WANT TO THINK ABOUT WHAT'S GOING ON UP THERE."

It may sound like a line out of a horror film, but the truth is we live in a world of constant stimulation and socialization. The only way to come out of it is with intentionality. Being alone with your thoughts requires that you be present with yourself. It requires much of what we discussed in Chapter 1 such as knowing yourself and subsequently liking yourself. Some people don't like who they are, so they spend every waking moment creating and living in this false reality. Oftentimes, this false reality presents itself in those who desire to be like another person so much that they begin to emulate that person in every way including that person's dress, mannerisms, public persona, etc. In a lot of the cases, these individuals have lost themselves in an alternate reality of being someone else. Instead of finding fear from your thoughts, take solace in the blessing that you have the opportunity to dive into a person who is wonderfully made with lots to offer in terms of energy, inspiration, and testimony.

In order to tell your story, you have to KNOW your story. Meditation acts as a chain breaker because it can free you from the very thoughts you're trying to avoid. Jack Kornfield wrote about conquering this perfectly in his statement from *The Wise Heart: A Guide to the Universal Teachings of Buddhist Psychology*. He wrote:

> Unhealthy thoughts can chain us to the past. We can, however, change our destructive thoughts in the present. Through mindfulness training, you can recognize those thoughts as what they are, bad habits we can recognize them as bad habits learned long ago. Then, we can take the critical next step. We can discover how these obsessive thoughts cover our grief, insecurity, and loneliness. As we gradually learn to tolerate these underlying energies, we can reduce their pull. Fear can be transformed into presence and excitement. Confusion can open up into interest. Uncertainty can become a gateway to surprise. And unworthiness can lead us to dignity.

His explanation serves as a tool to help us learn how to channel our energy in a positive way in terms of our feelings and emotions. This is the key to changing our perspective not only on how we view life but also how we live it. Allow your fear to be transformed into positive energies that resonate within and through you.

3. "I'M NOT DOING IT RIGHT."

There is no right and wrong way to meditate. Seriously! It's also safe to say that every meditative experience may yield something new, so they may not all be the same either. That's the beauty in it though, right? After all, we are habitual creatures, and we live our lives in this continuum of habits (some good and some bad). It's nice to let go of what is expected and simply be present in the moment to encounter each moment with freshness. With every moment comes a new experience. We look deeply into this moment and then let go as we move into the next moment without holding on to the previous moments. There is so much to be seen, learned, and understood along this path, and to rush it is to miss it. At that point, you've fallen back into a habit and are simply going through the motions. We sometimes can get caught up in asking ourselves, "Is this what I'm supposed to feel or see right now?" Don't worry about what you're "supposed to feel." Instead, honor your own experience in the moment. There is only one you with your DNA and your journey. There is nothing wrong with your journey. In fact, there is everything "right" with it. Don't look for an authority of any kind to bless your experience. Enjoy the journey moment by moment knowing it is right because it is authentically you.

4. "MY MIND IS TOO SCATTERED... I WON'T GET ANY-THING OUT OF IT."

If I asked 100 people in a room if their minds ever rested, I might see about 35% of them raise their hands. If I asked 100 women in a room if their minds ever rested, I imagine that percentage would decrease significantly to about 8-10%. I think women everywhere can attest to multitasking at its greatest. Does anyone else seem like they have a perpetual "TO DO" list? I feel like it never ends! Even though I'm a lover of lists and sticky notes (just so that I can cross the completed ones off for some sense of accomplishment), it never really ends. In full disclosure, sometimes it's a bit of a sock drawer up there. Everything is rattling around with no clear direction or home, so I'm not exempt either. Show me a person who doesn't have a scattered mind, at least sometimes. I'll wait...Exactly.

It's amazing that we will place preconceived notions on something that we've never even tried before. It becomes an excuse. Here is a little wisdom nugget to eradicate that thought from your vocabulary. LET GO! "Let go of what?," you ask. Let go of preconceived notions and expectations. According to Fadel Zeidan, Ph.D. (a neurobiologist and Assoc. Director of the UCSD Center for Mindfulness), "These subsequently lead to emotions that act as blocks and distractions." The remedy is simple. Try not to have any. Don't expect to experience bliss. Don't even expect to feel better. Remember when I talked about being in the moment? Just say, "I'm going to dedicate the next 5 to 20 minutes to mindful meditation," and then honor that commitment to yourself. The key to letting go is to continue to let go throughout meditation and thereafter. Zeidan continued, "During meditation, as feelings arise – annoyance, boredom, even happiness – let go of them because even they are distractors from the present moment," Zeidan added, "You're becoming attached to that emotional feeling whether it's positive or negative. The idea is to stay neutral and objective." Emotions can be distractions especially when their sole purpose or action is to calm the mind. Emotions can be like a busy street in the middle of the city. Nothing can get through, which leaves you stagnant. Letting go is a way to reduce the clutter and pave a way through it all to get to your destination.

You can choose options that will aid you in shifting your focus back to the present moment like returning to the changing sensations of your breath, returning to a mantra/chant, visualizing a particular image, etc. Just know that awareness of your busy mind is a part of the practice. On top of that, the mind wandering is just as natural as breathing. It's inevitable; the mind WILL roam during meditation. You may notice other sensations in your body or things happening around you, or you simply may get lost in thought while you daydream about the past or present or possibly judge yourself or others. All of this is OK. When this happens, simply notice what it is you were thinking about or what was distracting you. Then, take a moment to pause, acknowledge it, and let it go. You don't need to pull your attention right back to your focal point of choice. Instead, let go of whatever it was you were thinking about, re-open your attention, then, gently return your awareness to your focus. Then, guess what? Your mind invariably will wander again. Don't beat yourself up about this; it's natural, and it's a part of the practice. Remember, it is not THAT it happens. It is about how we respond WHEN it happens because it WILL happen. Whatever comes, acknowledge your thought without ascribing too much judgement to it and without allowing it to carry you away into exponential thoughts. Take a moment to come back to the present and resume your meditation. There is work and growth in the practice of meditation. It's your journey. Enjoy it from moment to moment.

5. "I DON'T HAVE ENOUGH DISCIPLINE TO STICK WITH IT."

Discipline! Ahhh, it is one of my favorite and sometimes most challenging words. Merriam Webster defines discipline this way. Discipline is the ability "to train to do something in a controlled and habitual way." It also can be described as an "activity or experience that provides mental or physical training." That definition fits too, doesn't it? There are some people who know themselves enough to say they struggle with discipline. There are others that simply choose not to talk about it. However, the above statement goes back to what I said in the third statement. You can't make an assumption about something to which you've never given enough effort. The truth is that if you are meditating, you are achieving success. There is no answer key to meditating. You simply take your journey one moment at a time.

What makes us disciplined at certain things is our ability, passion, habitual nature, or existential need to do it. We can change the above statement by changing the narrative that goes along with it. Meditation is tough because it falls out of your normal routine, so make it a part of your normal routine. Like our routine of showering and brushing our teeth, carve out time specifically for your meditation. Meditation is a mental and a spiritual exercise. Just like physical exercise, you may run into mistaken assumptions, unrealistic expectations, self-judgement, and the worst one, the tendency to quit. To hone your discipline, you must place meditation on a level with eating and bathing.

Time is a prized commodity for us all, but we make time for what we think is important. If you are struggling with the inability to focus, unhappiness, lacking purpose, frustration, depressed moods, etc., meditation IS INDEED VERY IMPORTANT. Your life (quality of life) depends on it. Make meditation a priority so that you do it daily. Now, of course, life situations will get in the way. Just like anything else, if you run into a lapse of a week or more, simply make the effort to continue it regularly. The first few days may or may not be the most challenging. Remember that Rome wasn't built in a day, and you weren't either. You don't expect to jump up and run 10 miles after a long hiatus in your exercise/jogging routine so don't come into meditation with expectations either. Simply show up and work through each moment as it comes. That is your success.

MY GLOW UP

We shouldn't stop being mindful when we stop meditating. The purpose of mindfulness meditation is to become mindful throughout all parts of our lives so that we're awake, present, and open hearted in everything we do. Mindfulness meditation aids in you making decisions and choices that are beneficial to you. "No" shouldn't be a foreign word to you, and "Yes" shouldn't be the only word you know. It's all about balance. When you are mindful and aware, you are able to live unapologetically and free without a lot of regrets. I didn't say, "without any regrets." It's natural to have some, but you'll find the majority of your choices and actions are what you desire from your heart and nowhere else.

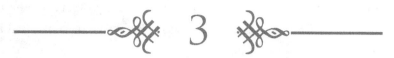

COMMUNICATION: DECODING THE MESSAGES (BRAIN ⇌ BODY)

I remember when I was younger, my mom put me in piano lessons. I loved music, but practicing the piano as much as I should…well, that proved to be a little more challenging. Nonetheless, I'd practice long hours in preparation for my piano solo performance. No matter how many recitals I played in, on performance day, I felt AWFUL. As the person preceding me was nearing the end of his or her solo, I'd proceed to talk myself down off the cliff because I felt like whatever I had for lunch might not make it through my digestive system. I would sweat profusely and would have that general ill-feeling. Even though it never happened, I'd feel the impending need to vomit. It was horrible, but I'd push through it, and as soon as it was over, all of those feelings would go away.

I'm sure many can identify with what I was feeling as a little girl before my piano recitals. All too often, we feel similar feelings in our adult life on a daily basis. For instance, the mother who is excellent in most things and tends to be everything to everyone (family, work colleagues, community, etc.) always seems to feel exhausted and tired. She works 8 to 10-hour days, exercises 5 days a week, eats a balanced and nutritional diet, and even sleeps 8 hours nightly. Yet, her most persistent feelings are, "For me to be so healthy, why am I always so tired? I just don't feel like I can make any headway."

Have you ever experienced either of the scenarios I described? Perhaps, you can identify with both of them. Many of us do. The first thing to note is there is a direct correlation between an emotional and physical response. This is known as psychosomaticism. So, let's define it and identify the role it plays in your life daily. Merriam Webster defines psychosomaticism as relating to the interaction between the body and the mind; It also is a physical illness or other condition caused or aggravated by a mental factor such as internal conflict or stress.

When you're angry, do you realize certain physical signs and symptoms that appear? Do you recognize these signs and symptoms when you're sad? Happy? Excited? Determined? The list could go on. If you've never taken the time to note or pay attention to your body that closely, I encourage you to not only receive what I say but also experience it for yourself. Our body is constantly sending and receiving messages through the nervous system. Here's a quick neuroanatomy lesson. Our nervous system has various components, but the primary portion is known as the central nervous system (CNS). The CNS encompasses the brain and spinal cord. The spinal cord connects to every nerve in our body, and our nerves relay messages to and from the brain which acts as a relay station. It tells our heart to beat, our stomach to digest, our legs to move, and our lungs to breathe. In chiropractic, we call the flow of this power "above, down, inside, out" because the information flows from the brain ABOVE the spinal cord, DOWN the spine, and from the nerves INSIDE that flow OUTward to our tissues, organs, and various systems within the body.

If we were to look at our spine, we would see these oddly square shaped bones (vertebrae), and in between them are gelatinous shock absorbers we call intervertebral discs. The spinal cord runs through a hole in the center of the vertebrae and extends out of additional openings in the bone; there are nerves that exit the spinal cord at each level. Think of it this way. An air traffic control tower (our brain) sends a constant flow of messages (nerve signals) from the planes in the sky (our body) to the tower and vice versa. That process allows our airline transportation industry to operate safely and effectively. If something were to happen to the signals between the tower and the planes, that would be a dire and dangerous situation. Therefore, when we have disruptions in our nerve signals, they manifest as stiffness, aches, pains, high blood pressure, diabetes, disease, etc.

The spine is the relay station or the switchboard. The brain is the central computer, and the nerves are the roads by which the nerve signals travel to get to their various destinations. These signals govern everything we do in our body. For instance, in order for me to pick up a sheet of paper, my eyes see the paper, and my brain interprets and creates the message. This message/signal travels down my spinal cord to the level(s) that controls the movement of my arm and hand in the cervical (neck) region. In a sense, the body sends a completion message from the arm/hand up through the spine to the brain once that action has been completed. On more than one occasion, I've had some of my patients ask questions like, "If the signals are flowing, what can possibly cause interference in our nervous system? What creates these traffic jams that cause dysfunction in our body?"

Nerve interference is caused by the three T's: trauma, toxicity, and thoughts. Our physical causes of trauma can come from small repetitive stresses called microtraumas. A microtrauma is a very slight injury that often goes unnoticed. The damage of microtraumas is that they are cumulative. It's not the first time, second time, third, fourth, or fifth time, but at some point, the accumulation of small injuries will result in a larger injury. For example, ladies, we tend to carry our purse on the same shoulder, or men tend to sit on their wallet as it rests in their back pocket frequently. This can lead to shoulder injuries and hip dysfunction over time. We also can have large macrotraumas like car accidents, falls, athletic injuries, etc. which cause immediate damage and injury.

Toxicity comes from the chemical stresses found in the air we breathe, the food we eat, and the things we drink (or lack thereof), etc. How many of us eat and breathe the perfect air and the cleanest food ALL the time? It's pretty challenging to do that since we don't have control over a lot of those essentials like air, soil, water, etc. If you've ever had the opportunity to visit one of the islands in the Caribbean then one of the things you may notice immediately is how clean and fresh most of the food is that you may eat. Due to the lack of excessive industrialization, their soil tends to still hold a lot of its nutrients. They eat off of the land and shop in markets with fresh deliveries as opposed to large grocery store chains. The air is clean because it blows off the ocean and the waters of the sea tend to be of a beautiful crystal clear blue hue. (I just made you want to hop on a flight didn't I?) The toxicity in the body is often directly correlated to what we consume.

Lastly, we have emotional stresses, which I'm sure none of us ever have, right? The stress you encounter in your daily routine from getting the kids off to school, meeting deadlines at work, and even getting along with every person we meet (kids and spouse included), can cause interference in our body which affects our health and our energy. The stress of your thoughts interferes with the message transmission that takes place in our nervous system.

Again, the question becomes, "How do you clear the traffic jams?" Well, that's what this book is all about. It is about helping YOU to be the emergency team that responds and gets things cleared for traffic to flow smoothly again. It takes work, but if you're reading this book, then you're ready to work. Understanding what the messages are helps us to decode them. You can only fix what you can identify. I'll say that one more time for the people in the back. You can only FIX what you can identify. Once you are able to interpret that your back pain isn't necessarily coming from a dysfunction in your spine because it is the byproduct of the anger you feel towards someone, you can take the appropriate steps to rid yourself of your emotional and physical pain and get back to living your best life. The exact cause for the evolution of a psychosomatic disorder or its symptoms is unknown; however, in keeping with the mind-body connection theme, physical disorders associated with mental stress are due to the hyperactivity of the nerve impulses sent from the brain. These signals alert the body and trigger a stress response which releases adrenaline into the blood that is exhibited as anxiousness. This condition can be triggered by various life factors including biological irregularities (i.e. glucose metabolism alterations and irregular amino acid levels), stress influence (i.e. trauma, abuse, illness, and frequent negative emotional disruption), and family circumstances (i.e. parental absence, relationship difficulties, or abnormal behavioral parent-to-child interaction).

Psychosomatic illness can be categorized into three types. In the first category, a person has both mental and physical illness, and the symptoms and management of the symptoms complicate each other. For example, a patient has bipolar disorder as well as hypothyroidism. The treatments are different and likely may include adverse drug reactions. Have you listened to a pharmaceutical commercial lately? There are a million and one side effects that you may experience to treat one symptom or condition. Now, imagine having two conditions or more. The second category involves a person who experiences mental issues due to the medical condition and its treatment. For example, a patient feels depressed because he/she has cancer and is taking treatment for it.

The third type of psychosomatic illnesses is called somatoform disorder. This is a condition in which a person with mental illness experiences one or more physical symptoms even if he/she does not have any associated medical condition. Some of the most common somatoform illnesses include hypochondriasis (believing a minor physical symptom to be a grave disease. For example, a person gets a headache and automatically panics thinking it's brain cancer), body dysmorphic disorder (People feel stress about the appearance of their body such as wrinkles or obesity and those feelings lead them to subsequent disorders on the other end of the spectrum like anorexia and cosmetic surgery addiction), and pain disorder (People sense severe pain over any part of the body which lasts for months or years without any physical cause).

An example of the pain disorder includes migraines, tension headaches, back pain, gastrointestinal issues, etc. Unfortunately, most of us have fit into at least one of the above categories at some point in our lives. Have you ever wondered why your back pain just doesn't go away or why you constantly get headaches a few times a month with no physical cause to your knowledge?

Increased psychosomatic symptoms worsen when people repress their emotions. There are some people who don't express their emotions, but instead, they hold them inside. Do you know anyone who might fit this description? This repression of their emotions can be especially harmful to their physical health. One study showed that people who repress their emotions are more likely to have disruptions in the normal balance of the stress hormone, cortisol, compared to people who freely express their emotion. The consequences of a hormonal imbalance over time from chronic psychological stress likely change the way the body functions at a hormonal and immunological level. Your hormones regulate the function of your body systems and your immunity provides protection against foreign invaders and dysfunctions in the body. When these systems are impaired, the body becomes vulnerable to a buildup of by-products that can be harmful to the system which contributes to the development and progression of cancer and cardiovascular disease from the abundance of free radicals in our system. Free radicals are, put simply, the by-products of cellular processes that cause damage to cells, proteins, and even your DNA.

Remember the three T's? Your thoughts (i.e. psychological stress) are connected directly to your mental state. If these stressors aren't properly addressed, the reality is what you believe can lead to disease and even death. I don't want to sound morbid, and I certainly don't want to scare you, but it's true! Due to the mind-body connection, the way you think and feel contributes to your physiological state of health or disease. If you do not explore and deal with painful emotions, they can create an underlying sense of anxiety, depression, or anger that physically can disrupt the body's natural ability to heal itself. This leaves the body vulnerable to an abundance of free radicals that cause damage. Without the ability to heal itself, the body can be susceptible to many diseases including cardiovascular disease, cancer, diabetes, etc. Contrary to what most people may believe, pain isn't just physical. Pain is essentially the combination of the physical sensations you experience, the emotions you feel, and the meaning the pain has for you.

Physiologically speaking, emotional suffering, physical pain, and other sensations share similarities in their neural pathways. For example, feelings of anger or insecurity can disrupt the regular beating of the heart and the calm flow of the breath. This further activates the sympathetic nervous system or the fight or flight system in the same way that it is disrupted when you are facing a threat. This interruption creates an even greater sense of unease and pain. As a result, the body releases hormones from the adrenal glands atop the kidneys to help the body cope. This can lead to adrenal fatigue or a mild form of adrenal insufficiency resulting from chronic stress and the body's inability to keep pace with the demands of perpetual fight or flight activation. Signs and symptoms include hair loss, exhaustion, depression, lightheadedness, hyperpigmentation (skin discoloration), fatigue, body aches, and unexplained weight loss, just to name a few. This condition is commonly apparent in those individuals with chronic stress and a lack of social support. They are more likely to have cardiovascular and other health problems than those with consistent and supportive relationships.

Another example of the powerful link between the mind and body is the fact that decreasing symptoms of depression may improve survival rates in cancer. This is why one of the primary parts of cancer treatment focuses on having a good support system to help share, shift, and pass the stress and angst to someone you love so they can carry or discard it while you focus on the fight of your life. Psychological support is important to deal with emotions and changing beliefs. It can help reduce depressive symptoms as well as inflammation in the body while bridging the gap in emotional and social support as it relates to the mind-body connection.

Cancer is something that has touched each of our lives in some way. While some of the battle is physical, most of it is metaphysical, a combination of the emotional and mental components of the individual. Studies have shown that positivity is just as important as the physical medicines that people take during treatment. It's the will to live and overcome that has led to millions of people to be able to walk as survivors in spite of the various cancers that run through our communities. This reality exists no matter where you are. On a smaller scale, even minor emotional stresses can set off smaller psychosomatic mind and body symptoms such as colds, viruses, back pain, and allergies. Interpreting these minor stressors negatively or feeling powerless against them makes us vulnerable to suffering from them.

To understand the mind-body connection, it's important also to understand how our current medical system plays a role in it. Mainstream medicine and its theories on infectious disease are based on the germ theory expressed in the 1860s by Louis Pasteur. Current theory based on Pasteur's ideas says that when specific microbes (germs, bacteria, viruses, cancer cells) enter the body, they produce a specific disease. This theory, however, neither considers the role of consciousness in this process nor accounts for how it affects the way the immune system responds to those microbes or the role stress plays on the body as a whole.

Unlike mind-body medicine, conventional allopathic medicine ignores the mind-body connection and uses chemotherapy, radiation, antibiotics, antivirals, and other drugs to attack and destroy these organisms. Conventional allopathic medicine purports that if there are no microbes left, there will be no disease. This commonly held belief suggests that our health can only be restored if germs or microbes that cause illness or disease are eradicated. This is only partially true. Pasteur later changed his own theory to include more influence from the environment or external factors, to include consciousness. Pasteur's theory has been the premise of our Western medical system to date. Please don't misunderstand my stance. Know that I am a believer in the medical system because it saves lives, however there is another aspect of health that governs the collective unit of the body, and that is the health to which I ascribe.

I spent years in the allopathic system and witnessed the good and the bad of it. Thus, my conclusion includes identifying the cause of the disease (metaphysical, consciousness, etc.) for elimination as opposed to the exclusion of such influences and focusing solely on the body. The reality is that we are constantly exposed to germs, bacteria, viruses, and we even have a certain number of cancer cells in our body. The outdated germ theory does not explain why these cells multiply at one time and not another. Furthermore, treatment ONLY with medications does not tap into our internal holistic healing power that our body is self-healing and self-regulating within the right environment; it temporarily corrects the surface problem and reinforces the concept that the healing power is external. In a perfect world, we have a sense of balance in which the medications and surgeries work in partnership with the mind-body self-healing techniques as we search for the internal emotional blocks to heal the real cause of disease. Reconnecting yourself with the mind-body connection that exists within you means that you've paid attention to the messages in your body and taken a stance to search for the internal emotional blocks that may be at the root of your ailment. This mind-body connection often leads to a decreased reliance on medications. Furthermore, this same connection serves as the ultimate demonstration of your self-healing ability. This connection will help you make better choices that will increase the probability that your health will improve.

In the end, decoding the messages from your brain to/from your body requires it to get all three systems on the same page to speak the same language. You don't want your body to be like the descendants of Noah in the Biblical reference of the Tower of Babel who attempted to build a stairway to Heaven to be like God so that they wouldn't need Him. No one spoke the same language which created pure chaos and little progress. Of course, the importance of this story is much bigger because none of us can be like God. We always will need Him, and He is always there for us no matter what. My reference for this Biblical account is to reinforce the idea that we don't want to be like those people. We don't want our body, mind, and spirit to speak different languages so that we fall into this tailspin of constant exhaustion, a depressed spirit, and an existence void of vibrancy. Not only do we want to be able to interpret the messages, but also we want to respond to the messages for increased quality and quantity of life.

My GLOW Up

We are all simply a series of connections as neurological synapses that transport and translate messages continually from our conception to our death. We don't know what we don't know because we haven't been introduced or educated enough about ourselves to recognize, correct, and improve the decoded messages/signals. When we ignore the messages and signals we receive from our brain and/or body, we live unilateral lives with signal notifications on mute. Unmute them all and land on the same page so you can speak the same language. THEN, listen to understand what your body and brain need to live symbiotically and whole.

CHAPTER

4

CREATING A SPIRITUAL SANCTUARY

Have you ever seen the migraine commercials? Perhaps worse than that, have you ever LIVED the commercial in which the mom is sitting there while the kids are screaming, playing, and running everywhere? The baby is crying. The phone is ringing. The husband is talking, and she just looks like she wants to disappear. If you're watching the cinematography like I am, they zoom in for a close up of her agony as they talk about the wonder drug, and suddenly, everything ceases a bit. It ceases at least long enough for her head to stop swimming and for her to become functional again.

I've been that woman in the commercial. Maybe, I haven't been her so much in the literal sense, but definitely, I have been her in the sense of everything happening at once and wanting to crawl into a silent dark hole to attempt to sleep off the craziness in my head. It's a miserable feeling, and those who suffer or have suffered from migraines assuredly can identify with that feeling. Did you know that many migraines are stress-induced or at the very least, have stress as the true culprit? I can attest to their true debilitation as there have been many days when I made it home, only by God's grace, crashed on the bed, and wallowed in agony until I was able to fall asleep. That is misery I wouldn't wish upon any man. We will discuss creating a spiritual sanctuary for the sake of saving you from at least most migraines you have yet to experience in your future.

Many consider a spiritual sanctuary to be the church, a temple, a synagogue, etc. However, your spiritual sanctuary is what you make it. It's a place of peace where you are able to sit and collect your thoughts, dream your dreams, and reflect on your life. It doesn't have to look a particular way. It simply has to serve you in the capacity of what you need and desire of it. Therefore, ask yourself, do you currently have a spiritual sanctuary? When you think of this place, does it evoke a sense of peace and restoration? Is this place easily accessible? These are the questions you must ask yourself when creating your space. There are two types of spiritual sanctuaries we can have...correction, we should have. The first type is that space in your mind and heart where you find rest. The second type is a physical location where you can dwell and find rest. We will explore how to erect both of these vital spaces so that you can have a place of refuge when needed.

In that commercial described above, usually the "wonder drug" (as I like to call it) is a magic pill that makes it all go away so that life can be new again. Full disclosure, some of them actually work...really well, but they come with hefty side effects. This chapter and this journey isn't about a "wonder drug," or perhaps it is. You see, this journey will allow you to create your very own "wonder drug" inside yourself first and then translate it outside of yourself to a uniquely created space just for you.

In that commercial, what they did portray was the drug as her safe space. You can create your own safe space, sphere, or cocoon of safety and silence wherever you are, and you don't need a drug to do it. This place should be somewhere where only you and God reside, which makes it a very intimate space. The vehicle to this space is meditation, and the driver is you. The idea behind your sacred space is to replenish your spirit. Living in a day in which you're very easily pulled in a million directions, your sacred space will serve as your time to reconnect with you, reconnect with God, and embrace everything you are to you. We sometimes tend to live in a world where we give everything, and we become what we are TO everyone else instead of taking the necessary time to embrace life and simply be present in who we are to ourselves at our core when no one is watching, and no one is present.

We get sucked into titles and oftentimes allow those titles to define who we are. This causes us to lose ourselves. You'll find yourself saying things like, "I'm a mother. I'm a wife. I'm a doctor. I'm a lawyer. I'm a teacher. I'm a student. I'm a caregiver." Your identifying statement should really be, "I am ME. I'm not what I do or who I am." Creating this sacred space does that. You may wonder, "How do I go about creating my sacred space?" Well, you must spend some time thinking about what makes a space sacred for you. This can differ for every person. You may find it helpful to set an intention before setting out along this thought journey. Don't allow the word "intention" to throw you. Though it may not be a word that frequents your vocabulary (unless you practice yoga), we set intentions all of the time. The most common time we set them is New Year's Eve. You set intentions for what you want to cultivate in the coming new year. You now have a word for what a majority of people in the world do around the time when a new year is beginning.

Setting an intention simply means choosing something that you want to amplify or cultivate in your space and in your life. It will help you create more clarity in your life especially when you plant the seed right before you begin your meditative practice. Think of setting an intention as drawing a map of where you wish to go. It becomes your driving force to help you become a better you and be present in each moment to live life with fullness and peace. People often use intentions with the practice of yoga. You are going to use it to create your sacred space mentally so that you can create your sacred space physically. The exercise for this chapter consists of two parts. The first part includes writing a list of intentions down on a sheet of paper. I'm a big fan of writing simply because it engages more of your senses. You think it, write it, and read it with your eyes, and you read it aloud and hear it with your ears. It's tangible because it rests on a sheet of paper. It seals it into your consciousness. I personally used this principle through school, (bachelor's level, master's level, and doctoral level) and it's successful and proven.

In setting your intention, think of WHAT you want to manifest and HOW you want to FEEL in the process of creating it. Sarah Prout lists 7 steps in setting powerful intentions. Let's explore these seven. As you follow along in your Transformation Guide, I have provided a space after each step where you can fill in what that step looks like *for you*. Like I said at the beginning, this is a manual of sorts to find and start the process of becoming the best version of yourself. It doesn't end when the book ends, and that's the beauty of it. It's ever-changing and evolving. These exercises will morph as you do. I wrote this book with the hope that you can come back and read it over and over for a new revelation. Each time you read it, I hope you discover something different about yourself. With that being said, let's begin.

1. **Create a Ritual**

   Most people have a ritual already and don't realize it. For example, New Year's Eve is a great example of a ritual. That's why the gyms are packed, farmer's markets and grocery stores are bustling with people, and people have set their various intentions for what they want to happen in the new year. This doesn't have to be the only time though that you make intentions. I find myself setting intentions at multiple points throughout the year. I'm always on a path to be better. My husband joins me in this practice, and we make it a family affair.

   To really get to the heart of what YOU want, you want to be comfortable and relaxed in your environment. Maybe, that means curling up on the couch with a blanket and a cup of tea. It might mean sitting on the beach with the crashing of the waves as your soundtrack. It could be as simple as sitting in the bathtub with a candle lit and a glass of wine. Whatever your favorite place is, that's where you want to aim to go. Your ritual should be personal and unique to how you love to do things. Therefore, this process looks different for everyone. That also means there is no right and wrong way. There is only your way and your ritual which will leave you inspired, uplifted, and ready to journey through and to your process of greatness.

2. Be Specific

While we may sometimes live in a world of generalities, the essence of who you are is VERY specific. Thus, when setting your intentions for the specific and uniquely awesome person you are, you also must BE SPECIFIC. I'm specific in most things that have to do with me. When I pray, I am particularly specific in my requests, thankfulness, and reverence to God. Specificity creates connection. It requires you to dive deeper to share and explore more of who you are such as your needs and your desires. The difference is huge. For example, if you are trying to prepare dinner for your someone special, and you ask, "Honey, tonight I will cook whatever you want. What does your palate desire?" If the person's answer is, "Chicken is fine." That doesn't give you a whole lot to go on, does it? You then have to ask questions like, "How do you want it cooked? What sides would you like to have with it? Do you want dessert?" At that point, it kind of loses its vibrancy, right? Whereas, it would be much clearer for you if the person's response was, "I'd love the basil and garlic seared chicken you make with mashed potatoes and kale greens and maybe birthday cake gelato for dessert." Now, if I can choose, the second response would be my choice!" See? Specifics alleviate the guesswork. It works the same way when you set your intentions. You want clarity with your intentions and goals, so they must be specific.

3. Get Creative

Try to think outside the box. Sometimes we have a tendency to limit ourselves to what we see, what is common, and what is expected. I'd like for you to be creative and daring enough to think from a place of unlimited abundance. Think from a place with no ceilings or walls. It should be a place where your wildest dreams can become a reality. Don't assume that things are impossible. Everything was once considered impossible, but it took someone with a wild and crazy intention or idea and the vision and fortitude to make the impossible possible. This is what I want for you.

4. Allow Yourself To Dream

As you pick up from where you left off in the third step, I want you to allow yourself to dream. Allow yourself to dream on an entirely new level than where you reside ordinarily. Think about the things that radically could change your life forever. What are they? What would it take to make those things a reality? What are the action steps required? As you dream, eliminate all limits and boundaries. Some might say, "The sky is the limit." I say there is no limit. It doesn't matter where you begin. It only matters where you're going and what you're dreaming.

5. Get Into the Feeling Space

I'm reminded of the lyrics of a James Brown's song that said, "I've got the feeling, baby baby. I've got the feeling." I want you to feel. Get into the feeling space and feel...everything, anything. We live in a world where people are afraid to feel. As a result of everything being bottled up, chaos ensues. Depression and misery run rampant in our society because the emphasis isn't placed on feeling; the emphasis is placed on portraying greatness as opposed to embodying greatness. People find that it's easier to live in a false reality than it is to live in and improve the real one. We discussed in earlier chapters that your thoughts are directly connected and working in conjunction with your feelings. When you get into the feeling space along with the intentions you create, you also manifest those things as you journey through the process of what your intention really means to you. Imagine what you would feel if you are in the moment when you've already manifested your desires. You have to start or begin with the end in mind. Take that feeling and allow it to inspire and fuel your process as you progress to achieve your goal. The process is equally as important if not more important than arriving at your intention or goal. Feel the abundance that awaits you. Feel the love that surrounds you. Feel the creativity that pours out of you. Feel the love that IS you.

6. Let It Go

The phrase, "Let It Go," can be a whole series of books in itself. Once you've set your intentions (process and all), you must let them go. If you hold on to them, they cannot take flight. Letting go may be the hardest part of the process, but it is a necessary step. You need to let them go to get out of your own way. If you don't, you easily fall victim to distractions. Distractions affect everyone. They come in like little mites and eat away at intentions, hopes, and dreams. They can create roadblocks in the intention-setting process by diverting your attention to things that don't matter in that present moment. Can you identify some of your distractions? Identifying them is the first step in your journey to wellness.

7. Reflect With Gratitude

The last part of this process is reflection. Reflection serves two purposes. The first is to look back to the beginning and give thanks for reaching or achieving your intention or goal. The second purpose, which I think is the most provocative one, is to reflect on the process and everything you learned along the way. In my opinion, it is here where your growth takes flight. Reflection is by definition an effect produced by an influence (i.e. your intention and goal). The reflection is the effect your journey has had in becoming who you are today. Reflection requires that you reconnect with yourself. It requires that you reconnect with the feelings you had at each stage of your intention setting, and it creates humility in your experience.

Now that we understand intention, you should have a greater understanding of why it's so important to DO so when creating your sacred space. You can ask yourself the following questions before creating your space. What are you seeking to add to your life by setting this space apart in your home? What do you hope to do in this space? How will you honor God in this space? How often do you see yourself using this space? Everyday? Important holy days? Seasons? Who will share your space with you? Will you allow your partner to take part in creating it and using it? Will you include your children at times? If so, is the space safe for him or her? Once your space is created, it should evoke a sense of peace prompting you to feel that call and commitment to do the work every time you pass it. Creating a sacred space isn't something done in secret. It is often helpful to include your partner and family in the discussion of why you need to have this space and what it means to you. When those closest to you understand what you need, their support simply fuels the journey to self-awareness and peace that radiates from inside of you outwardly to those you love and cherish.

When you are seeking a space, you want the area to be peaceful and uncluttered. It should be separate from where you work or pay bills and away from kids playing and lots of traffic. If free space is limited, get creative to optimize the space. Look for corners of the room that aren't being used. Once you find a space, add a partition, curtain, or screen for privacy and separation. Find something that meshes with your sense of style and evokes a spirit of calm within the space. This could be something like a windowsill or nook. You even can use a bookshelf or dresser to hold the objects that calm you while you occupy the space on the floor or the bed. You can use objects to make your space sacred such as a beautiful pillow or a special blanket that you include in your quiet times and moments of meditation. You even can create a portable sacred box filled with unique items that are meaningful to you. This way, you create your sacred space wherever you are based upon the sacred items you have with you.

When you are setting up your space, use all of your senses to evoke feelings of peace and tranquility. Think of things that you love to touch, hear, taste, see, and smell. You can include candles, music, pictures, affirmations, and items of various textures, colors, etc. You also can include inspirational items to place in your space such as a vision board, plants, devotional items, religious books, Divine inspired tools, incense, essential oils, etc. Incorporating the use of a journal in your space also helps you keep a list of your intentions, desires, and blessings. Try to spend time in your space every day. Make it a practice of removing your shoes when you enter your sanctuary. Removing your shoes and changing into comfortable clothes creates separation and vulnerability in the space. This space should invoke a feeling of freedom which includes being free from the restrictions, stress, and weight of the external world. This space is reserved just for you. It's clean, quiet, and peaceful. Once your space is created, please note that it may not stay the same. In fact, it shouldn't remain the same. As you grow and evolve, your sacred space will change.

MY GLOW UP

Detaching and disconnecting is a real thing. It's healthy. It's the place where introverts (like me) live and breathe! It's also a place in which extroverts have difficulty finding peace or relaxing. What it does is re-establish the connection to ourselves that easily may have gotten lost in the hustle and bustle of daily living and interacting with others. Create your space and use your meaningful items to help you stay connected to yourself for a renewal of your spirit and be reminded of the peace that exists within you. Imagine going into each day with peace and a smile no matter what the circumstances are that you face.

EAT, *PRAY*, BREATHE, LOVE...
LOVE LANGUAGE TO GOD

Growing up, I remember listening to the radio and hearing gospel artist, Shirley Caesar, tell the story, "I had a praying grandmother...and because of that I knew enough to call on the name of Jesus." Going to Sunday School and church every Sunday and walking into my mom's room on many occasions and finding her on her knees at her bedside, I was very aware of prayer. My mom not only took me to church, but also she emulated and modeled what prayer and being a child of God looked like in our home, family, and community. She gave me my foundation of knowing about Christ and who He was. I gave my life to Him at a young age, and while I wasn't perfect by far, I, too, knew enough to call on the name of Jesus because I had a praying mother and grandmother who kept me covered and governed in Christ.

As a result of that upbringing, I know the value of prayer. Of course, there were parts of it that I didn't understand fully until I matured and got older, but my foundation was solid. In time, I found out WHY prayer was the crux of my family, faith, and foundation. When I needed answers and guidance to life's situations, sometimes, the only answer that would suffice was the one coming from my Creator, Christ Jesus.

The first question that should be answered is "What is prayer?" Prayer is simply an active form of communication to God. The passive form of prayer can be executed in the act of meditation. Prayer is our direct line to Christ...no switchboards, no hold times, and no busy signals. The line is always open, and He always answers. God desires for us to communicate with Him all the time. In our society, we have every device known to man to help us communicate from landlines, cell phones, and bluetooth devices to computers, chatrooms, social media platforms, and video conferencing. All of this, to some, may seem complicated, and I would agree. If you've never had any experience with technology, it can be a daunting experience. To many people, prayer seems complicated. Prayer is simply talking to God in the simplest way. Let's explore the logistics of prayer with scriptural references.

The two most common questions people ask are, "What do I say?" and "How do I say it?" What you say is whatever you want. It's like talking to your best friend! It's easy to talk to someone when you know he or she loves you unconditionally! That means that no matter what you do, that person's love for you will never cease. The closest we come to sharing this form of love is when you are a parent. You have unconditional love for your children even when they stray, disappoint you, or separate themselves from you. A parent's love is sustained through all of that. How much more is the love Christ has for us? Can you imagine parental love to the infinite power? NO MATTER WHAT, God's love for us never wavers, and it's never predicated on what we do or don't do. We sin, but He still loves us. We don't love ourselves, and He still loves us. He ALWAYS loves you, and that should make it easier to talk to Him because He cares more about you than you care about yourself. What do you say when you want to talk to God? You can say anything you want, but here are three launching points/examples to help you start:

1. Ask Jesus to forgive you of your sins and make you new in Him!
   "Now turn from your sins and turn to God, so you can be cleansed of your sins." Acts 3:19

2. Tell Him your needs, wants, desires! Don't carry worry, give it to Him!
   "Give all of your worries and cares to God, for He cares about what happens to you." 1 Peter 5:7

3. Thank Him! There is so much to be thankful for, and He gave us all of it. He died so that we can live, so thanking Him for his sacrifice is our duty.
   "For God so loved the world that He gave his only Son, so that everyone who believes in Him will not perish but have eternal life."

The second question is, "How do you say what you say?" The answer to that is simple. You say it with confidence, joy, and expectation. When it comes to Christ, He is our number one cheerleader and supporter.

1. We communicate with Christ with confidence and the belief that He will deliver. Why? Because His Word tells us so.
   "Because of Christ and our faith in Him, we can now come fearlessly into God's presence, assured of his glad welcome." Ephesians 3:12
   "So let us come boldly to the throne of our gracious God. There we will receive his mercy, and we will find grace to help us when we need it." Hebrews 4:16

2. We communicate with Christ with joy because we know He can deliver.
   "You have shown me the way of life, and you will give me wonderful joy in your presence." Acts 2:28

3. We communicate with Christ with the expectation that He will deliver.
   "Listen to my voice in the morning, Lord. Each morning I bring my requests to you and wait expectantly" Psalm 5:3

"I am praying to you because I know you will answer, O God. Bend down and listen as I pray" Psalm 17:6

This is our foundation of prayer. In getting to know yourself, who better to ask than the One who created you. Prayer is not just meant for us though. We should pray for others. Many times, the ones closest to your heart cause the most stress for you. Of course, it's not intentional on their part. That's just how life is. We shouldn't carry these worries; we should submit them to God in prayer. Jesus set the example for this in the Bible when He prayed for His disciples and for every generation to come that would follow Him. His prayer was that God would protect and strengthen them as long as they are in this world. Does that sound like a prayer that you could pray for your family member or for your friend? Jesus didn't stop there. He also prayed for those who would come to believe in Him through the gospel message. That means that He prayed for the unbelievers in your life, or if you are an unbeliever, Jesus prayed for you. (John 17)

Prayer is the unifying piece which contributes to our knowledge of ourselves. When we pray, we also should pray with faith. Faith is knowing God will do things for us even when it seems impossible. God lives in spirit. Our faith helps us to believe in this God who we cannot see or touch. However, through prayer, our connection with Him grows, and we are able to feel Him, hear Him, and see Him all around us. We grow in faith, love, and knowledge as we spend time with Him. (Hebrews 11:6) As a result of our knowledge and connection with Christ, we should pray with worship and reverence. He is a God who sees all and knows all. He is holy, mighty, and worthy of praise and exaltation. (Psalm 99:5 and John 9:38)

The Bible is full of encouraging scriptures for prayer that will aid in our growth and understanding of who Christ is and subsequently who you are. (Philippians 1:9) Ultimately, if you don't know how to pray, God loves us so much that He left us with a template to follow until we gain the confidence to talk to Him. It is called the Lord's Prayer, and it is found in Matthew 6:9-13.

The Lord's Prayer (Matthew 6:9-13)
"Our Father in heaven, hallowed be your name,
your kingdom come, your will be done,
on earth as it is in heaven.
Give us this day our daily bread.
And forgive us our debts, as we forgive our debtors.
And lead us not into temptation, but deliver us from evil.
For Yours is the kingdom and the power and the glory forever.
Amen."

If you feel led, say this simple prayer below.
God, I love you. I ask your forgiveness for the things I've done that have dis-
appointed you, and I pray that you change my heart and my mind so that I am
able to stand in confidence with you. I may not find comfort in you always or
know how to talk to you, but I ask you now for your help in leading me to you
for reliance and comfort. Help me to grow in the knowledge of myself and how
you've created me. Teach me how to love myself and others. Teach me how to pray
and have faith in the destiny you have for me. In Jesus's name, I pray. Amen.

MY GLOW UP

Having the fundamentals of prayer instilled in me from childhood made it easier to make active those principles and valued lessons I needed for the purpose of peace of mind and survival later on. There simply are some problems man cannot fix. Advice is wonderful, but knowing when to change the source of your advice is the key to alleviating depression, frustration, and ultimately, disconnection. We've been talking a lot about connection, connection with yourself, and now connection with God. Establishing a two-way connection reminds you that you are never alone in this world. He's with you daily. Not having a foundation doesn't mean you're lost. It simply means that you have to establish one. How do you do it? You simply have a conversation with God like you are talking to anyone else. No fancy, overly spiritual language is necessary. Just chat, anytime, anywhere.

PART 2

MENTALLY: MIND OVER MATTER

CHAPTER

6

WHAT IS STRESS?

As both a doctor and a prior respiratory therapist, I've got stories for days from my experiences in the ER, various ICUs, rehabilitation facilities, long term care facilities, private practice, etc. Check out these two scenarios because there's a question coming in a bit that will require you to answer it. A man enters the ER with labored breathing, tightness in his chest, sweaty palms, and a tension headache. After all of the tests are done, the results are inconclusive. There is no physical reason why this man feels like he is having a heart attack, yet he declares he is. He's diagnosed with anxiety, given something to calm his nerves, and sent home. Unbeknownst to the medical staff, this man has just been laid off from his job of 8 years due to company downsizing. His wife has just given birth to their brand new baby girl which made them a family of 6. They have one child in high school preparing for college, a teenage girl who is looking forward to prom like other girls her age, and a son who loves to play every sport known to man. They've recently purchased their dream home in the past year, and to add insult to injury, it's coming up on Christmas.

This might be what you call stress. This gentleman is experiencing stress in all facets of his life: physically, mentally, and emotionally. Thankfully, we can assume that his high dose stress is only temporary.

While you may not have this situation in particular, we all have stories that if we had enough time to hear them all would yield varying degrees of stress. The key is to keep an awareness about what's happening so that you can make appropriate changes swiftly to remedy the stresses and embrace peace.

Stress is a phrase coined by Hans Selye in 1936 who defined it as the non-specific response of the human body to any demand for change. It also can reflect the body's reaction to any change that requires an adjustment or response. The body can react with physical, mental, and/or emotional responses. Stress is considered a normal part of life; however, how you handle stress can be detrimental to your health and psyche if you allow it to harm you. You can experience stress from your environment, your body, or your thoughts, and it is manifested physically, emotionally, or mentally.

According to the American Psychological Association, there are three major types of stress, acute stress, episodic acute stress, and chronic stress.

The first type is acute stress. It's the most common form, and it comes from demands and pressures of the recent past and anticipated demands and pressures of the near future. In small doses, acute stress can be thrilling and exciting, but too much can be exhausting. An example of acute stress is a challenging ski slope that is exhilarating early in the day. However, if you let a few hours pass and try to conquer that same ski slope later in the evening, your experience can have the opposite effect which is both taxing and wearing on the body. Skiing beyond your limits can cause fatigue which results in injuries and broken bones. Likewise, acute stress in abundance can lead to psychological distress, tension headaches, upset stomach, and other symptoms. Acute stress is most commonly caused by the daily trials of life like an isolated issue at work, a sick child at home from school, a flat tire, or a missed deadline. Due to its short-term status, it doesn't have enough time to do extensive damage to the body. As a result, it likely will manifest itself as symptoms in one or more of the four following categories:

- Emotional distress is generally a combination of the three stress emotions: anger or irritability, anxiety, and depression.
- Muscular problems and body aches include tension headache, back pain, jaw pain, and pains associated with pulled muscles, tendons, and ligaments.
- Digestive system issues affecting the stomach, gut, and bowel, including heartburn, acid reflux, flatulence, diarrhea, constipation, and irritable bowel syndrome.
- Other symptoms mainly related to our adrenal glands that lead to elevation of the blood pressure, rapid heartbeat, sweaty palms, heart palpitations, dizziness, migraine headaches, cold hands and feet, shortness of breath, and chest pain.

The great part about acute stress is that most of these symptoms are readily identifiable as stress-related. Acknowledging your stress is the first step to alleviating it.

The second type of stress is episodic acute stress. These are simply individuals who suffer acute stress so frequently that their lives are reminiscent of an episode of the game, Twister, because they are full of chaos and crisis. Typically, they are always in a rush but are also always late. Newton's law generally applies to their lives because if something can go wrong, it will. They tend to take on too much and overload their plates. They can't organize the overwhelming demands and pressures fighting for their attention. Seemingly, they are perpetually in acute stress with no end in sight. Episodic acute stress manifests itself as individuals who are often over-aroused, short-tempered, irritable, anxious, or intense.

When you are talking to them, they may often give a self-description of having a lot of nervous energy. You may see them pulling or chewing their hair, shaking a leg, fidgeting, etc. Another form of episodic acute stress comes from worrying excessively. Have you ever had someone in your life who just worried about everything? These individuals tend to see disaster around every corner and live life as pessimists. They tend to be more anxious and depressed than they are angry and hostile. The symptoms of episodic acute distress include persistent tension headaches, migraines, hypertension, chest pain, and heart disease. Due to the level of symptomatology, the interventions in place for them occur at a number of different levels and generally take many months. They may have lifestyle and personality issues such as blaming their issues on other people. They also struggle with external events that make them fiercely resistant to change.

Chronic stress it's the last type of stress. While acute stress can be thrilling and exciting, chronic stress is not. This is the long-term stress. This is the grinding stress that wears people away day after day, year after year. Chronic stress is the stress that destroys bodies, minds, and lives. Put simply, it wreaks havoc through long-term attrition and the breakdown of who you are. Chronic stress tends to result from the stress of finances, dysfunctional families, an unhappy marriage, a despised job or career, etc. It simply comes when a person never sees a way out of a miserable situation. It's the stress of unyielding demands and pressures over an insurmountable amount of time. These individuals simply give up searching for solutions. Chronic stress also can stem from traumatic early childhood experiences that become internalized which causes them to remain painful and present. Some of these experiences can have profound effects on people's personalities or deep-seated convictions and beliefs. The worst aspect of chronic stress, however, is that people simply tend to get used to it. They forget it's there, and thus, it becomes a silent killer that dismantles the body piece by piece. Plainly stated, it simply becomes familiar and comfortable. When you hear the phrase "stress kills," this is the stress to which they are referring. This stress kills through suicide, violence, heart attack, stroke, and perhaps even cancer.

According to the U.S. Stress Statistics by the American Psychological Association (APA, 2017), an overwhelming 77% of people regularly experience physical symptoms caused by stress. 76% of people cited money and work as leading causes of their stress, and 73% of people regularly experience psychological symptoms caused by stress. Stress is linked to six of the leading causes of death: heart disease, cancer, lung ailments, accident, cirrhosis of the liver, and suicide. It is important to note that chronic stress can wear down the body's natural defenses leading to a variety of physical symptoms including dizziness, aches and pains, grinding teeth, headaches, indigestion, increase in or loss of appetite leading to weight gain or weight loss, problems sleeping, fatigue, exhaustion, sexual difficulties, etc. What exactly happens in the body when we are stressed? Let's explore the physiology of stress.

When stressed, the body thinks it is under attack and switches to fight or flight mode. This mode causes the body to release a complex mix of hormones and chemicals such as adrenaline, cortisol, and norepinephrine. This complex cocktail prepares the body for physical action by causing a number of reactions from diverting blood to the muscles to shutting down unnecessary bodily functions such as digestion. Fight or flight mode refers to the way the body reacts in cases of stress. Often used alongside the example of the caveman preparing either to fight the tiger or run away, what happens in the body to fight the tiger is the heart pounding, an increase in his breathing rate, the shunting of blood from his heart to his extremities, the dilation of his pupils to see the environment surrounding him better, and the ability to focus his attention so he is able to respond quickly to the situation. Whether the caveman chooses to fight or to give flight and run away, the body prepares to encounter additional stress by making these physiological changes.

Have you ever been scared or startled? I remember, one day my Mom and I had come home a little early and we decided jokingly to scare my bonus dad. Now, he was a very gentle and kind man. To know him was to love him. He had a prior military history in which he served and spent some time in the Philippines. There, he learned and became quite proficient in one of the martial arts. My mom came around the corner, and all we heard was "Whhhhhhhhhhhaaaaa..." He took his opening defensive stance before realizing it was us. He jokingly coined the phrase, "throw hands," and said that's exactly what he was about to do. Needless to say, that was the first and last time either of us tried to sneak up on him. Why did I share this fond memory with you? Well, it's because in that moment, his stress system was activated, and upon hearing his warning of impending harm our stress systems also activated which included sweating, increased heart rate, dilated pupils, etc. Something like this is short-lived though. Once the moment passes, homeostasis begins to help the body regulate back to a normal and unstressed state under ordinary circumstances.

The issue is when our body goes into a state of stress due to inappropriate and longer-than-designed situations. If our blood flow is shunted to the most important muscles needed to fight or flee, our brain function is minimized. This can lead to our inability to think clearly and rationally which impacts both the home and work environments. If the body remains in this state of stress for an increased period of time, it can be detrimental to your health and result in elevated cortisol levels which can increase your sugar and blood pressure levels and decrease your libido. Lastly, stress also can cause us to freeze. For some people, prolonged stress sets the stage for dysregulation. The energy mobilized by the perceived threat gets locked into the nervous system, and we freeze. The most common symptomatology is holding the breath. In this state of stress, individuals often hold their breath and experience shallow breathing. The occasional deep sigh is the nervous system's way of playing catch-up on its oxygen intake.

Hans Selye hypothesized that stress affects the whole body, and it manifests itself as a sum of changes or a syndrome and not by simply one change. He called this the General Stress Syndrome. There are three components to the General Stress Syndrome: the alarm stage, the stage of resistance, and the exhaustion stage. The alarm stage represents a mobilization of the body's defensive forces as it preps for the fight or flight syndrome. Again, this involves a number of hormones and chemicals excreted at high levels as well as an increase in heart rate, blood pressure, respirations, perspiration, etc. The second phase is the stage of resistance. This stage occurs when the body becomes adapted to the challenge and begins to resist it. How long the body resists is dependent upon the body's innate adaptation energy reserves and the intensity of the stressor. The final stage is the exhaustion stage in which the organism enters and then dies because it has used up its resources of adaptation energy. Thankfully, few people ever get here. Scientifically, stress diseases are caused primarily by errors in the body's general adaptation process. This means that as long as the body's regulatory systems are functioning appropriately, the body is able to maintain balance and health. What causes the general stress syndrome is excess deficiency or disequilibrium in the amount of the body's adaptive hormones.

This chapter's exercise focuses on you acknowledging what stress feels like in your own body. Refer to Experience 2.1. in your participant workbook.

MY GLOW UP

Two of the most important things to know about stress are the signs and symptoms. You can't fix what you can't see. The moral of the story is to be vigilant about how your body feels and how you feel. Adapting to a feeling of dysfunction does not equal functionality. It is important to remember that we never were designed to operate in a constant state of stress. The body simply tires, and after a while, it stops functioning in its optimal state. This affects weight fluctuations, hair loss, memory, immunity, energy, muscle and joint pain, headaches, etc. It ultimately can lead to system failure, so it's important to pay attention to your body's response to stress.

CHAPTER
7

GOOD STRESS VS. BAD STRESS; IS THERE A DIFFERENCE?

In a matter of months, I went from living life and dating pretty cool people (none of which were my match really even though I met them on Match.com) to being introduced to and reluctantly set up blindly with someone that led to a long distance relationship, a proposal, the planning of a wedding, the purchase of a home, and instant mommie-hood. I am one of those people who can tout having a whirlwind romance! I never saw that happening, but it did! My husband is amazing, and thankfully, we met at a point in our lives when we lived a little, experienced a lot, and played no games about expectations, wishes, deal breakers, and desires. I experienced a lot of good stress that at times transitioned to periods of bad stress. When that happened, I had to decide to stop and take a breath and a break. This period was probably one of the most exhilarating times of my life, and within a blink, it was over. As I planned the wedding of my dreams with the man God sent to me with as much peace in my heart as one could have, I knew I was blessed. Perhaps, I even could be the display of too blessed to be stressed because in spite of all the bad stresses that came along with this event in my life, none of them destroyed the goodness that was happening. If I had a meltdown (and there was ONE), it quickly turned around when I realized that God loved me enough to bless me with all this goodness... pray, let go, and let God. That's what I did.

There is a myth that says all stress is bad. This is not true. There are such things as good stress and bad stress. Though we never hear someone say the words, "I'm feeling really stressed, and it's such a great feeling," the reality is that if we didn't have some stress in our lives (i.e. the good stress variety), we'd feel unhappy, unaccomplished, and stagnant. If we consider stress as anything that alters our homeostasis, good or bad, then good stress is pertinent for a healthy life. Wouldn't you agree? However, any good thing in overabundance can turn out to be not so good anymore. Therefore, too much good stress can turn into bad stress and vice versa (not a typo, the explanation is coming).

Psychologists refer to good stress as eustress. Eustress is the type of stress we feel when we are excited, exhilarated, and happy. Our hormones change, and our pulse quickens, but this change does not happen out of threat or fear but out of excitement. This is a type of stress we feel when we ride a rollercoaster, run for a promotion, or even go on a first date. One would think *if good stress is beneficial for me, then I should get as much of it as I can.* You don't want too much of this good thing though. You want to choose activities that are important to you that make you feel pleasant and excited about life. You also want to eliminate as many activities as you can that drain you or end up leading you down a path to chronic stress.

There's a quick exercise you can do to tell which activities truly are good for you and which ones can lead to your detriment. As you ponder each particular activity, pay attention to the thought and consider how it makes you feel. Do you feel excited at the thought of performing said activity? Is this an activity that you want to do or have to do? This is a really important question because it's easy to fall into the trap of doing things to make other people happy especially when you care about them. When you're deciding on an activity, make sure you really want to do it or decide if it's something that you've gone along with to appease someone else. If the latter is true, cut it. This is what I call setting priorities. Women, oftentimes, have the habit of putting themselves last. I've been guilty of this myself. You have to reach a point when you decide to choose yourself not only because you can, but also and most importantly, you choose yourself because you should.

Now, I want to explain how stress can change. Too much good stress can become bad stress, and bad stress sometimes can even become good stress. This sounds weirdly complicated, right? A good example of good stress becoming bad stress occurs when people experience it in excess like the manner in which adrenaline junkies live their lives. This phenomenon of good stress becoming bad stress is due largely to the fact that the body doesn't recognize the difference between good stress and bad stress. Your stress response is triggered either way. If you're adding that to pre-existing chronic stress and several other stressors, there's a cumulative effect which equates to lots of stress! This is why it's important to connect with yourself and be in tune with yourself to be able to tell when enough is enough. Eliminating all stress is farfetched, but there are often ways to minimize or avoid some of the stress in your life making the rest of the stress you have a little easier to handle. Getting rid of the largest mountain of stress makes the smaller amounts of stress more tolerable. This change in stress levels builds resistance in the body against the types of stress in your life that might be unavoidable.

On the opposite side, bad stress can become good stress, but not all forms of stress are eligible for this upgrade. The trick to this process is to change your perception of some of the stressors in your life. This shift in perception can change your experience of stress! The physiology behind this is that the body's stress response reacts strongly to a perceived threat. There is little difference physiologically in the response that your body generates to something that it perceives to be a stressor and a threat that is legitimate. If you don't perceive a particular stressor as a threat, the body doesn't trigger the stress response. Let's change the vocabulary a bit and shift our perception.

Instead of perceiving a stressor as a threat, let's instead perceive it as a challenge. When you do this, you turn fear into excitement and anticipate your success. Rising to a challenge also acts as a reminder of your strengths. Have you ever heard the phrase, "Perception is everything"? Well, it's a true statement. A pessimist tends to have thoughts fueled by negativity, fear, anxiety, and doom. If one is able to change his or her thinking from pessimism to optimism, that change generates feelings of positivity, hope, expectation, and excitement. We are creatures of habit, so the more you train yourself to turn your stresses into challenges, the more often your positive nature becomes automatic. People also achieve eustress by incorporating hobbies into their lives that promote goal setting and positive reinforcement.

Whether it's good stress or bad stress, did you know that stress can be contagious? I'm sure you did because I'm sure you've experienced it. Stress is tied intimately to our social world in which feelings of loneliness and isolation can take their toll on the brain and body. These forms of stress can lead to depression, anxiety, and heart disease. Stress doesn't have to affect your body and brain directly. It can affect you indirectly in the daily lives of your loved ones. This can be in the form of health problems that affect a loved one, family responsibilities, and relationship issues that lead to mental and physical health consequences for both of you and your loved ones. One source defines stress as a perceived disconnect between the situation and our resources to deal with the situation. Whether real or imagined, stress acts as a threat and taxes our resources. *See Experience 2.2 in your participant workbook.*

My GLOW Up

Ultimately, eustress will inspire and propel you to complete a given task or goal instead of allowing it to debilitate you. As a bonus, research has shown that eustress enhances and improves cognitive brain functioning, keeps the mind sharp, and maintains the good physical condition of the body. Though some stress is inevitable, it's negative effects on the brain and body don't have to be. By altering the way we interpret the world around us, we can gain control over stress, change our perception about a situation, and develop the power to see its benefits.

HOW TO PRIORITIZE STRESS

P icture this. We were three months post wedding, and my mom was going in for a transplant. My husband was laid off 2 weeks prior to our discovery that we were expecting our first child together. Unbeknownst to us, the next 9 months would be a faith walk and full-blown testimony. Here I was, pregnant and two steps from bed rest due to the lovely combination of fibroids and pregnancy. We were without a stable income for almost a year. My mom was in the fight of her life. Our finances were strained to say the least, and life was happening fast. Life was so fast in fact that our faith became our sustenance, and that's how we lived. Talk about high stress circumstances. Whew! Most people who know our testimony wonder HOW we survived and how we came out stronger than ever on the other side. I always say that it was ALL GOD because it was. I also will say that He dropped certain strategies in my spirit that allowed us to prioritize our stresses so that we did not get overwhelmed by the circumstances. Let's dive in so that I can show you how to do the same.

Stress will never go away. Our lives never will be completely stress-free because at the moment that occurs, we cease living. We've discussed eustress, good stress, and distress, bad stress. We win in life when we learn to avoid trying to rid our lives completely of stress and learn to prioritize our stress. Priority is defined as the fact or condition of being regarded or treated as more important than something else. Another definition is the right to take precedence or to proceed before others. Let's name some things that people commonly consider priorities. You are a priority. Your spouse and/or your children are priorities. Maintaining the household is a priority. Maintaining a spiritual connection or relationship may be a priority. Behind God, the next priority in terms of importance should be you. However, men and women alike often directly or indirectly choose to place themselves last. Why is that? Is it a lack of self-importance? Is it a lack of self-worth? Is it hero syndrome? Is it even intentional? Here's the reality that you face. While you may be an integral part or piece of a puzzle, your value does not exonerate you from prideful actions that lead to stress-induced outcomes. "Doc, what did you just say to me?" What I said was don't take on the world and sacrifice yourself.

People always will ask of you. It's just the way it is, but no one knows your limits like you do. Thus, it is your responsibility to make your limits known to your job, your community, your family, your church, your spouse, and your children. It's important to remember that you are a human being FIRST. When you came out of your mother's womb, you were a human being, and that came before all the roles that are commonly attached to you now. You first must be a healthy human in order to be a healthy wife and/or mom. You first must be a healthy human before you can be a healthy husband and/or dad. If you are continuously stressed and maxed out, how much of you are you *really* able to give to those you love most? How much of you are you really able to give to yourself? I like analogies, and this is one I often use.

We run like a car. When we're fueled up with a new pan of oil and fresh parts, the car runs well. Your fear of breaking down on the side of the road is virtually nonexistent. You even may find your peace and solitude in your car. What happens when the car no longer has any gas? I affectionately call this "running on fumes." You're in desperate need of an oil change, and you need new tires. What happens? We begin to stress about the condition of the car. Well, at least, I hope you do. Not only that, you also end up evaluating when you might be stranded on the side of the road with all of the angst that comes with that thought. Now, have you ever found that YOU are "running on fumes?" What do you do about it? Here is where most of us fail epically. Do you stop, refuel, take time to address the inside, and rework the outside or do you just keep riding that car until its demise?

If you've found that you don't stop and refuel, and you've actually admitted it, let me be the first to congratulate you on taking the first step. One of my many rules of life is, "You can't fix what you don't see." Meaning, if you can't be honest with yourself when you are strictly by yourself, when will you be honest? Many self-help organizations utilize this first step which is recognizing when you have a problem. You don't have to be addicted to drugs or alcohol to have a problem. We ALL have problems. In order for you to make any changes or progress, you must be honest with where you are and desire to move forward. Now, if you are among the growing number of individuals who finally are taking the first step out of pride and into humility to prioritize yourself first, you are now ready for the rest.

Raise your right hand and repeat after me, "I used to be Captain Save Everyone, but today, I choose me. Today, I will take at least 10 to 15 minutes to engage with myself. I am growing in my understanding of the importance of cultivating a healthier me. Today, I pledge to release my title and cape and return to being me...awesome, present, and growing."

Only when you are able to reach the point of needing help and most importantly receiving help can you grow and be the best you - the best mom or dad, the best wife or husband, the best daughter or son, the best colleague, and the best leader. We all should desire to lead by example. The questions I want you to answer are, "What example are you setting for your children as they watch you handle the world?" Are you stressing to them the value of self-care and self-preservation or are you pushing them to go, go, go until they drop? If you aren't teaching them to rest and recover, why aren't you? You see, in my profession, it is my job to ask you the difficult questions. I didn't seek to write this book for accolades. My passion for writing this book is to stimulate a change in those who read it. My passion is to stimulate a change in you. Therefore, my questions, my exercises, etc. are meant to challenge you. They are meant to prune you in an effort to spur you along the path of greatness that is both in you and that IS you.

You can't learn to prioritize stress until you prioritize you. I'll say that one more time for the ones in the back. You can't learn to prioritize stress until you prioritize you. Prioritizing stress is a way of preventing the feeling of being "maxed out" from stress overload. You can't handle everything at once. That's neither practical nor sensible. Just as if you were a student in a high-level math class working on a complex problem, you have to use the priority of functions in order to solve the problem correctly. The same is true for prioritizing your stresses. The same approach you'd use then is the same approach you'll use now. The only thing that's different is the topic. This topic literally can change your life. Step one in prioritizing your stress is to prioritize YOU.

Step two in the process is make a list, check it twice, and even include what's naughty and nice. (Do you see what I did there?) Make a list of your stressors and leave a few lines between each stressor where you can write something later. Don't assign a number to them just yet. I just want you to make the list first. Be sure to include EVERYTHING that stresses you on your list, good and bad. Why is step two to make a list? There is something about writing things down that is cathartic and therapeutic. It makes it real.

Once your list is complete, go back and label your stressors with a G (good) or a B (bad). Sometimes, with all that life throws at you, it's easy to become inundated with the bad stressors and lose track of all the good that is present in your life. By creating a list, you are able to recognize that there is good in your life. Your job is to learn to prioritize those stressors so that you can establish and/or recognize a healthy balance.

After labeling your stressors, I'd like for you to number your stressors. Think about the top 10-15 most important stressors in your life. They can include family, career, friends, etc.

Step three in the process is to acknowledge your list. What do I mean by that? Starting with the stressor labeled number 1, take AT LEAST 30 seconds to write down what makes this a stressor. For example, one of your stressors might be financial instability, so you might write that you're behind on your car payment, and bills outweigh your income. You want to be specific *without* going down a rabbit hole. Give 1-2 specific examples and then the general summation of the issue. After recording *why* it's a stressor, write 3 changes you can make to your current situation that can alleviate some of the pressure (distress) or increase more of the joy (eustress). We'll continue with our last example. Your three things might be to eat out less and cook more, reduce entertainment to small amounts on occasion (free whenever possible), and seek an additional part-time job for extra income. Use this approach with every item on your list from one to ten. When you bring awareness to your stressors, you are better able to approach them one by one. Remember that Rome wasn't built in a day, and you weren't either.

We are a sum total of our experiences, genetic tendencies, and environmental influences. You may not always be able to choose the environment you are in, but you can choose how you respond to it. One person can take the unfortunate circumstances of childhood neglect and abandonment and choose to travel the road that repeats that troubled past. Another individual with that same history can choose to take the road where he/she is determined to do better and be better while refusing to be a product of his or her environment. Therefore, as you assemble and dissect your list, you may find that some of your stressors stem from past experiences like childhood, previous relationships, etc. Diving deeper into each one of those experiences often provides you with a window of realization and change. As you progress through this exercise, you are creating your own blueprint for how to handle your individual stressors. The beauty is that you can return to this exercise over and over again as you evolve.

The final step is to take your changes and decide how you are going to implement them into your life. If you have 3 changes per stressor, that's at least 30 changes to make if you listed 10 stressors. That can be a lot all at once so take the first change of each stressor and write down how you plan on implementing that change into your daily life. Aim to implement a new wave of changes every 2-4 weeks. Ten changes may seem like a large number, but the idea is the good on your list will balance out the bad on the list. Nonetheless, if you feel like you need to break it up and implement five changes instead of ten, do that. Stretch yourself, but don't overdo it. Every step is a step in the right direction. Small successes lead to large gains. The key is to be consistent in your upward movement. Additionally, you can prioritize your stress by incorporating certain activities into your lifestyle to cultivate mental health and wellness. We'll discuss a few of my favorites.

#1: MAKE THE "SERENITY PRAYER" YOUR MANTRA

God, grant me the serenity to accept the things I cannot change, courage to change the things I can, and wisdom to know the difference.

The Serenity Prayer is often an instrument used in the rehabilitation support world to help those coping with internal and external stressors. If we learn to accept things like traffic, per say, and focus only on the things we can control, we win half of the battle. Mental anguish, labored breathing, and shouting expletives will NOT make those lanes of traffic move any faster. What you can do is turn on your favorite tunes (or if you're like me...your favorite book) or make your phone calls to let people know that there is traffic, and you will be arriving late. In essence, you must learn simply to go with the flow. My motto is always that stress never solves any problems; it does create them though.

#2: MY SECOND FAVORITE IS CLASSICALLY SIMPLE: REMIND YOURSELF TO BREATHE.

Did you know that when you are stressed, angry, or in pain, your essential capacity to breathe leaves you or is diminished greatly which affects your heart, brain, and body? As a result, you don't breathe or you take shallow breaths, and this change prevents the release of the stress, tension, or pain signals. We will dive into breathing in the next couple of chapters but taking intentional deep breaths to breathe *through* the tension instead of holding your breath which is essentially holding onto your tension is the goal and a key element in helping your body cope.

#3: SERVE OTHERS.

It's easy to get caught up in your own stresses and forget that others around you are dealing with stresses that are similar or different to the stresses that you are experiencing. A study in the American Journal of Public Health found that those individuals who'd gone through stressful events and went on to help others had a reduced risk of stress-related mortality or death (Poulin, 2013). The Bible says in Revelation 12:11 NIV, "They triumphed over him by the blood of the Lamb and by the word of their testimony; they did not love their lives so much as to shrink from death." Support is an essential component of life. John Donne wrote, "No man is an island, entire of itself; every man is a piece of the continent, a part of the main."(Donne, 1624). We are all connected as pieces of a puzzle. God placed gifts inside of each of us. As trials become testimonies, we are commanded not to hold onto them but to share them. Why? We are all a part of a bigger piece and larger realm of life. The next time you feel stressed, find someone who may need your help and serve him or her. Whether you know that individual personally or through a service organization, you just might find that helping someone else often relieves some or even all of the pressure and tension weighing on you.

#4: CREATE A DAILY MEDITATIVE PRACTICE.

You learned about the power and purpose of meditation in Section 1. Incorporating meditation into your daily lives may be the key to your sanity. I take mediation a step further and combine it with my prayer and study time. The Bible says in Joshua 1:8 NIV, "Keep this Book of the Law always on your lips; meditate on it day and night, so that you may be careful to do everything written in it. Then you will be prosperous and successful." Meditate on the Word and meditate to rest your mind. Both of these may surrender peace to you.

#5: YOU'VE GOT TO MOVE IT, MOVE IT!

While earning my doctoral degree, my orthopedics professor used to say, "You've got to move it, move it, so you don't lose it, lose it." It was catchy, and many of us put rhythm to it and applied it to various concepts in the course like frozen shoulder (or medically known as adhesive capsulitis), etc. While it applies to the physiological principles, it also applies to life. Have you ever been so incredibly stressed that you just had to go for a walk to collect yourself? I think the above phrase would apply to that situation also, don't you? Taking a nature walk is often therapeutic because you are inundated by God's beauty all around you. This natural beauty makes it nearly impossible to remain upset or stressed. I like to think of it as immersing myself in Him and all He has created. I almost feel closer to Him and further away from anything that may be troubling me at the time. I often combine this practice with walking meditation which encompasses meditating on the goodness of God and standing in admiration of His works and how He has blessed you. It's called creating intimacy with your Creator. It doesn't have to be in the form of a walk though. If you need a little additional energy pushed out of you then you can incorporate exercising at the gym, going for a run, or practicing yoga as a form of movement.

All of the above examples are ways to prioritize your stress. It's not an exhaustive list by far. You can add, subtract, and make your own list that is specific to you, your needs, and your desires. These solutions aren't meant to imply that stress will go away. There always will be stressors in your life. Instead, it's a way of prioritizing the good that is in you to distract from the bad that seemingly can take over your life. It's meant to remind you that there is so much more to life than stressing about things. When you stress, you can't live. I'm sure you can think of a few worry warts in your family. If you can, consider sharing what you've learned with them. Share this book with them or gift them their own copy in the spirit of giving and service. Reducing stress and learning how to channel it appropriately makes everyone happier. You don't have to take my word for it. Simply apply some of the principles you have learned, and then ask those around you whom you love if they have seen any changes in you. You might be surprised to find that without asking them, you feel differently because your perspective towards stress has shifted. You've shifted from being powerless and pessimistic to being empowered and positive.

I have included below scriptures in the Bible for times of adversity for the moments in which you feel sad or overwhelmed. Go to your sacred sanctuary and meditate on the scriptures God has given to us in the Manual of Life.

- **2 Corinthians 4:8-9**
  We are hard pressed on every side, but not crushed; perplexed, but not in despair; persecuted, but not abandoned; struck down, but not destroyed.
- *Proverbs 3: 4 - 6*
  Then you will win favor and a good name in the sight of God and man. Trust in the Lord with all your heart and lean not on your own

understanding; and all your ways submit to him, and he will make your paths straight.

- **Philippians 4: 12– 13**
  I know what it is to be in need, and I know what it is to have plenty. I have learned the secret of being content in any and every situation, whether well fed or hungry, whether living in plenty or in want. I can do all this through him who gives me strength.

- **1 Peter 5: 10**
  And the God of all Grace, who called you to his eternal glory in Christ, after you have suffered a little while, will himself restore you and make you strong, firm and steadfast.

- **Romans 8: 28**
  And we know that in all things God works for the good of those who love him, who have been called according to his purpose.

- **Joshua 1: 9– 10**
  Have I not commanded you? Be strong and courageous. Do not be afraid; do not be discouraged, for the Lord your God will be with you wherever you go. So Joshua ordered the officers of the people

- **John 14: 27– 28**
  Peace I leave with you; my peace I give you. I do not give to you as the world gives. Do not let your hearts be troubled and do not be afraid. You heard me say, I am going away and I am coming back to you. If you loved me, you would be glad that I am going to the father, for the father is greater than I.

- **Isaiah 26: 3– 4**
  You will keep in perfect peace those whose minds are steadfast, because they trust in you. Trust in the Lord forever, for the Lord, the Lord himself, is the Rock eternal.

- **Philippians 4: 6– 7**
  Do not be anxious about anything, but in every situation, by prayer and petition, with Thanksgiving, present your requests to God. And the peace of God, which transcends all understanding, will guard your hearts and your minds in Christ Jesus.

MY GLOW UP

It is paramount to understand your stressors and see them written and listed before you can do something to correct or alleviate them. If you skip this step, you may find yourself bouncing like a ping pong ball from one stressor to the other and missing out on the blessed life that you've been gifted to live. As believers, we often have this misconception that we aren't meant to have trials. The truth is if we are to be like Him, we have to be like ALL of Him. He endured trials, suffering, and sacrifices so that we might live in the abundance that He's granted. James 1:2-4 says "Consider it pure joy, my brothers and sisters, whenever you face trials of many kinds, because you know that the testing of your faith produces perseverance. Let perseverance finish its work so that you may be mature and complete, not lacking anything." Who you are today is a result of the trials you have endured. As you learn more, the idea is that you are more prepared to endure your trials and succeed.

IDENTIFYING YOUR STRESSORS: FAMILY, FINANCES, FUN, & FAITH

At one point last year, I had A LOT going on. I was a distance caregiver for my grandparents and local caregiver for my Mom. I was balancing a university teaching schedule, developing a budding brand, writing my book, and educating families which is my passion. It was mostly good stuff, but it was A LOT to digest. As I was preparing to head out to teach one of my classes one Monday morning, my husband asked me if I was stressed. He hadn't said much as he watched me make a list, and tackle each task, so his question was warranted. I answered with a simple, "Yes, maybe a little. I just need a moment to slow down and collect myself." I grabbed a piece of this moment in the car on the way to work, and I allocated the rest of the time for after I'd returned home only to put out more fires on the end-less list of things to do. I'll be the first to admit that I'm not immune to stress. I, too, have taken these exercises and tools and incorporated them into my life. I'm so confident that they work because I'm proof!

First, I was able to admit that I was indeed stressed. I wasn't "over the moon" stressed, but I was experiencing some angst due to being overwhelmed. Additionally, I was able to identify what things were stressful to me. I always say, "You can't fix what you don't see." *How* do you identify your stressors? We explored a few of these signs in the previous two chapters. According to the International Stress Management Association (2017), I have provided a list of signs that may be a little more subtle and common. These signs fall into one of four categories: psychological, emotional, physical, and behavioral.

Refer to Experience 2.4a in your *G.L.O.W. Rx Guide* to complete.

Psychological Signs:

- Inability to concentrate or make simple decisions
- Memory lapses
- Becoming rather vague
- Easily distracted
- Less intuitive and creative
- Worrying
- Negative Thinking
- Depression and Anxiety

Emotional Signs:

- Tearful
- Irritable
- Mood swings
- Extra sensitive to criticism
- Defensive
- Feeling out of control
- Lack of motivation
- Angry
- Frustrated
- Lack of confidence
- Lack of self-esteem

Physical Signs:

- Aches/pains
- Muscle tension
- Grinding teeth
- Frequent colds/infections
- Allergies/rashes/skin irritations
- Constipation/diarrhea/IBS
- Weight loss or gain
- Indigestion/heartburn/ulcers
- Dizziness/palpitations
- Hyperventilating/Panic attacks/nausea
- Physical tiredness/exhaustion
- Menstrual changes/loss of libido/sexual problems
- Heart problems/ high blood pressure

Behavioral Signs:

- No time for relaxation or pleasurable activities
- Prone to accidents, forgetfulness
- Increased reliance on alcohol, smoking, caffeine, recreational, or illegal drugs
- Becoming a workaholic
- Poor time management and/or poor standards of work
- Absenteeism
- Self-neglect/ Change in appearance
- Social withdrawal
- Relationship problems
- Insomnia or waking tired
- Reckless
- Aggressive/anger Outbursts
- Nervous
- Uncharacteristically lying

We are likely to feel stressed by personal situations that are un-expected, unpredictable, or just plain out of our control. People with type-A personalities who NEED control oftentimes find themselves on the verge of mental collapse and feel like they might unravel as they lose control over even the simplest tasks. How many times have we seen this play out in the media or with our loved ones? This is a huge component in knowing yourself. It's not enough to know you are this way and still allow it to destroy you. You must take the steps needed toward acknowledging and identifying your stressors so that you can learn to prioritize them. This knowledge will aid in minimizing the effects that the stress has on the mental, physical, emotional, spiritual, and behavioral aspects of you.

That is WHY you are here. You must identify the various signs of stress you find that you are demonstrating OR that those close to you have seen you demonstrating. If you're not sure, ask your spouse, children, friends, colleagues, etc. Sometimes, other people are able to see things about you better than you can. Actually, I implore you to ask them and refrain from getting mad when they answer you. Don't engage in an argument if you feel they are wrong about what they see. I assure you that they have no reason to lie to you. In fact, telling the truth may be their way of helping you recognize everything they see in you, especially what you don't see. Be sure to ask the right people in your life. I intentionally include those outside of family because everyone's family dynamic is different. There are those who can love you but always see you for who you were in the past when it may not be an accurate representation of who you currently are.

One thing to keep in mind is that most stresses are indeed personal. Not only that, most stressors are also habitual. Stress tends to repeat itself due to the sources from which it is derived. The most common areas of stress derivation are:

- Conflict with loved ones
- Childcare responsibilities

- Eldercare Responsibilities
- Social Support network
- Physical health conditions (injury, trauma, illness, and pain)
- Psychological health conditions (depression, anxiety, alcohol misuse)
- Financial concerns
- Losses
- Uncertainty/disappointment
- Conflicting demands
- Lack of appreciation or recognition
- Lack of a work-life balance

With each personal stressor you may want to think about some of these questions: Why does this feel stressful to me? Have I successfully experienced this stressor before in the past? The most important rule here is to BE HONEST. This is about your growth and your *progress* through the *process* of you getting to know every part of you, especially the parts of you that you don't like. Oftentimes, I've seen that when people don't like something about themselves, instead of acknowledging and addressing it, they tend to tuck it away and put on a façade to emulate someone they admire. THIS is NEITHER healthy NOR is it productive. It's important to understand that you must have some honest, self-reflective moments about yourself, your stress level, and the sources of your stress.

One of the most common sources of stress that people are ashamed that they feel and subsequently hide is stress from children. Children can be and often are a major source of stress from infancy into adulthood. That's a part of being a parent. No one is going to judge you for saying those words that are allowable in a safe space. If they do, give them what I call the "do you" shrug and continue on your own journey. Their opinion is irrelevant which leads me to another common source of stress, social comparison syndrome, or as my mom labels it, "Keeping up with the Joneses." Am I the only one who ever wondered who the

Joneses were and what made them so popular? Unfortunately, due to the explosion of social media, many people have fallen victim to the invisible competition to have the best life as reflected on social media. Anytime you put energy into being someone other than yourself, it is wasted energy…wasted valuable energy.

Knowing the source of your stressor is a huge step in learning how to manage and alleviate those various stressors in your life. It's not enough to identify them. You must identify the source as well. Correct or modify the source, and you possibly can modify or even eliminate that particular stressor altogether. At the very least, you can address how it affects you and how you will manage it moving forward.

My GLOW Up

There are some stressors you'll find that originate from sources that you can control. You can choose your environment. You can also choose the time in which you exist in a stressful environment. However, there are other situations and environments from which the escape is not so easy. This is where the ability to identify the source of your stressors becomes paramount. You also have to implement practices that will help you prioritize and manage your stresses. Like G.I. Joe, "Knowing is half the battle." Take what you now know and implement it one stressor at a time, one source at a time, and one step at a time. You owe it to yourself to do that.

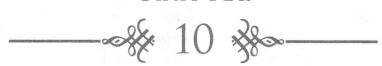

CHAPTER

10

EAT, PRAY, *BREATHE*, LOVE... PLACE THE "S" ON YOUR CHEST...FOR SUPER NOT STRESS

I remember when I was a respiratory therapist after graduating from college, I had a patient come into the ER with what we were trying to rule out as a myocardial infarction or heart attack. His symptoms were profuse sweating, chest pain, a racing heart, palpitations, labored breathing, lightheadedness, etc. To most people, a heart attack would be one of the first things to pop into their mind. The doctor came in after the staff ran a series of tests on the patient and told him it appeared as though he was perfectly healthy. The doctor followed with the question, "Have you experienced any stress lately?" The gentleman responded with a "yes" and began to rattle off a number of problems that included job loss, marital issues, mounting bills, and debt. He wrote him a script for anti-anxiety medicine and decided to discharge him, suggesting that he follow up with his primary care physician.

The gentleman described above is a prime example of what most people do when they are stressed. They either don't have an outlet or don't utilize one which enables stressors to mount and build until they explode or overflow in the form of a meltdown. This is what makes this chapter so important, I'm going to teach you or make suggestions of ways in which you can minimize the effects of stress. I have made the point in this book repeatedly that some stressors are just plain unavoidable. For those stressors, it's less about the stress and more about how you react to the stress, or better yet, how you're able to minimize the effects of the stress. No one is expecting you to walk around without a care in the world whistling while you work when all hell is breaking loose. No one is expecting you to don a leotard and a cape and fly all over with superhuman strength. That is NOT the expectation. The expectation is, however, that you will be able to respond to those various challenges with increased awareness of their negative effects so that you are left with minimal wounds and scars. Find that place in between and rock your unique SUPERpower(s). Replace the *Stress* on your chest with *SUPER* instead.

How often have you found yourself completely wigging out over something that was stressing you? Have you ever felt ill suddenly, and your actions just weren't a representation of who you are or who you are striving to be? Trust, it's happened to all of us. One of my favorite escapes I use to reconnect with myself in the middle of a stress storm is breathing. B-I-F stands for **B**reathing **I**s **F**undamental. Just like you can connect with yourself, you also can connect with your breath. This, in turn, connects us to our life. How do you do that? To connect with your breath, you will learn the art of pranayama. Pranayama is one of the seven limbs of yoga, and it bridges yoga, meditation, and breath awareness.

By nature, most people are shallow breathers. The exception is if you are an athlete or are very active on a consistent basis in your profession. Exertional movement (i.e. activity or exercise) requires a deeper recruitment of oxygen to the tissues by way of breath. Do you know how to assess whether you are a shallow breather like the masses? Sit still and monitor your breath. If you notice that the lower portion of your ribs barely move, even if you have movement of your abdomen, you are guilty of shallow breathing. Another indicator is the number of times you yawn. Yawning is the body's way of demanding and commanding more oxygen to be delivered to the brain. The correlation between yawning, being tired, and your breath is that when you're tired, you tend to do the bare minimum both consciously and subconsciously. Your body chooses to reduce the energy to draw in the necessary amount of oxygen. This leads to shallow breathing, which subsequently leads to a deficit that requires your body to push for a burst of oxygen it gains from yawning. It's a standard supply and demand or cause and effect relationship dynamic.

First, let's look at the physiological importance of breathing. What exactly happens when we breathe? The primary function of breathing is to obtain oxygen for use by the body's cells and tissues and eliminate carbon dioxide waste produced by those same cells. Breathing involves the diaphragm, lungs, and the pathways leading to the lungs starting from the nose and mouth and moving down the pharynx and trachea into the bronchi, bronchioles, and alveoli. Breathing is the ultimate endurance workout. The muscles that play a vital role in breathing are located near the lungs and are responsible for helping your lungs expand and contract. These muscles are the diaphragm, abdominal muscles, and intercostal muscles (muscles between the ribs), and those muscles in the neck near your collarbone. The lungs and blood vessels, on the other hand, are responsible for bringing oxygen into your body and removing carbon dioxide with the help of other portions of the airways listed above.

You really may not care about the importance of the physiology of breathing, but I'm a firm believer in knowing your body so you can tell when something is simply not right. When it comes to stress and pain, the breath is generally the first to go. Think about moments when you've stubbed your toe or slammed your finger in a car door. The first thing you may notice when reflecting on these moments is that you immediately held your breath and shook the appendage that you seemingly just lit up. Without going into a long explanation of neuropathophysiology and endocrinology, the short version of this explanatory hypothesis is that holding your breath increases blood pressure, which, in turn, reduces nervous system sensitivity and translates as a reduced perception of pain.

Now, I am going to remind you how to breathe. You once knew how to do it properly, but sometimes, as we live, and life happens, we forget how to breathe *properly*. Here's a simple exercise to help you improve or relearn diaphragmatic breathing. You can do this in a seated or supine position of laying on your back.

1. Either lie on your back or sit in a comfortable position with your knees bent.
2. With hands open and flat, place one hand (superior) on your upper chest and the other hand (inferior) below your ribcage resting softly on your belly.
3. Inhale slowly through your nose. Feel your abdomen expand as it presses into your inferior hand. Be sure to keep the superior hand still.
4. Hold your breath for a count of 1-2 seconds and exhale through your mouth with pursed lips. As you exhale, engage your core muscles (the most familiar muscles being those rock hard abs) of your abdomen drawing them up and back diagonally toward your spine.
5. Again, keep the superior hand on the chest still.
6. Repeat for the allotted time for your breathing exercise.

I recommend this breathing practice for 5-10 minutes per session at least 3-4 times daily. Ways to challenge yourself:

- Perform the breathing exercise with a book on your abdomen to add a small amount of resistance.
- Incorporate breathing exercises with varying degrees of activity.

Changing your approach to stress doesn't stop at breathing although it certainly helps. Other ways you can change your condition of being stressed to super include other aspects of self-care and self-pride. Here are just a few of my favorites that you can use IMMEDIATELY.

1. Attitude is everything! Have you ever heard of the age-old expression, "You get more flies with honey than you do with vinegar"? My family both taught and demonstrated this principle growing up. How you treat others is a direct derivation of your attitude. Have you ever been in contact with someone who had a bad attitude? In your observations, how did that person's attitude influence how he or she handled stress? Keeping a positive attitude is imperative to minimizing your stresses. It has a direct correlation to your reactions to certain situations. For example, if you ordered something and received the wrong item, a person with a bad attitude probably would get into a heated conversation with customer service and demand to be able to return the item or receive a substitute item. Additionally, that person's blood pressure likely would be elevated, and he or she would have a change in his or her disposition. A positive attitude would not only keep your heart from racing and blood pressure from spiking, but also it potentially could earn you a 20% discount on your next order or a refund AND reissuing of the order for the inconvenience. How you handle your stress often can influence others to respond in a different manner or follow in your steps so keep a positive attitude.

2. In line with keeping a good attitude when encountering stress, it's also important to be assertive instead of aggressive. Being assertive helps others listen and maybe even understand your feelings, beliefs, and opinions. Oftentimes, when stress is combined with a bad attitude, the resulting response is to become angry, defensive, depressed, or passive. Sometimes, it's even helpful to assert how you desire to feel so that your actions can

follow. Don't be afraid to guide your own emotions and actions with your words FIRST. You're worth it.

3. Another way to curtail a negative response to stress is by invoking the Serenity Prayer. "God, grant me the serenity to accept the things I cannot change, Courage to change the things I can, and wisdom to know the difference." Where most people fail is that last clause. Who am I kidding? The whole thing gets us caught up. That's the process of life. Part of effectively managing stress is accepting that there ALWAYS WILL be events that you CANNOT control. Creating a negative response to this reality does NOT change this reality. India Arie had a song that said, "Strength, courage, and wisdom has been inside of me all along." The key to living a life that is positive and productive is your ability to tap into these three attributes to apply them to various life circumstances and situations.

4. Incorporating a healthy lifestyle can change how you respond to certain stressful events. This includes nutrition, fitness and activity, meditation and yoga, and a support system. Studies show that when you eat well, remain active in fitness, and engage in social balance, you tend to feel better. When you feel better, you tend to be happier. With increased happiness comes the ability to incorporate the three actions above effectively.

Learning to manage your stress effectively is a test of endurance. You have to make a consistent effort and challenge yourself to change your own approach to life's circumstances, which will add years to your life and save you from the effects of stress. There are many things that can add an "S" to your chest. You get to choose what the "S" represents. Don't let stress be one of them. Make your life "Super" and not "Stressed."

My GLOW Up

Even though you aren't always able to manage your circumstances effectively, the one constant is that you ALWAYS can manage you. Understand that life WILL happen, but you WILL survive. Ninety percent of the impact of stress is how you respond to it so think before you act and remember that you are more than a conqueror. Stand up, stand strong, and act like what you are...a WARRIOR!

PART 3

PHYSICALLY: HEALTH FROM THE INSIDE OUT

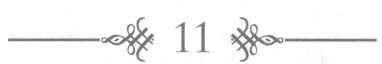

WHAT IS HEALTH?

I t's November, and Thanksgiving is around the corner. Christmas will be here before you know it, and the new buzz word is "health." Everyone wants to get healthy for the new year. It's the standard story. What do you do? You spend money on gym memberships, participate in health challenges, decide to go vegan or vegetarian, cut out meat and dairy, etc. You make lots of lofty promises that aren't always the easiest to follow through on *successfully*. Most times, by the time you make it to the end of the first quarter, you're back to your old habits, and nothing has changed (if you're lucky). With that, the stress and disappointment of not reaching your goals begins to weigh heavily on you, and you run the risk of becoming less active and eating less healthily, yet again.

I had a friend who used to fall inevitably into a cycle of little change and revert to those same old habits year after year. She had a definition of health, but it wasn't one specific to her. She found herself doing all of the "right" things according to the latest fitness or nutrition craze gracing the markets at the time. She wanted to lose weight, and she tried it ALL...literally. She exercised and changed her diet. You name it; she did it and only found that she became more and more unhealthy and depressed than she was before she made the change. She had no consistency, no direction, and no guidance. Her only focus was the new hot thing. She jumped from diet to diet and fitness program to fitness program until she decided to stop and slow down long enough to understand what health meant for her. Once she took this time, things began to change in a positive direction for her. She made some realistic dietary changes that she was able to maintain, her activity level increased, and she was able to have better quality sleep and more meaningful engagement in her relationships. Oh! AND she lost weight and hit some of her target weight goals she had been trying to hit for years. She was happier, and it showed!

Let's first look at the definition of health. Health is defined by Webster's Dictionary as the condition of being sound in mind, body, and spirit; free from disease; and a flourishing condition of well-being. Here is a quick pop quiz. If I presented to you the scenario of a 34-year-old young woman who after eating dinner one evening found herself running a fever and vomiting profusely, would you say that she was healthy or sick? Try this one, a 50-year-old father of 3 decided to play basketball with his kids for a few hours on a Saturday afternoon after they'd made the request a dozen times. Would you say that he is healthy or sick? Now, the common misconception is that health is the absence of symptoms and pain, but I would like to provide you with more information. That 50-year-old father who actually smokes a pack of cigarettes a day has lung cancer unbeknownst to him and doesn't know it because he "feels fine." Now, that 34-year old young woman felt ill because she ingested food that wasn't cooked appropriately and was poisonous to her system. The fever was her body's way of increasing the temperature of the environment so that bacteria wouldn't survive long enough to affect her organs long term. The vomiting was her body's way of getting rid of the bacteria expeditiously. Now that you have that information, let's try this quiz again. Is the 34-year old woman healthy or sick? How about the 50-year old father? If you answered *healthy* and *sick* respectively, then you are correct!

While we all desire to be healthy, it is of the utmost importance that you establish a TRUE definition of health and redefine what that looks like for you. To do so requires a strong constitution. Health, as defined by the media and corporations, is often very different from the foundational concept of health. There is no one-size-fits-all approach to anything, especially your body. Peer pressure and comparison play a role in most people's false definition of health with things like "body goals." We try to look like or attain the body imagery on social media and depicted by celebrity personalities. Why do we do this? I think it's simply because there is a lack of a full understanding of what health is and what it is not.

There are certain habits science has proven to contribute positively to health. Habits like working out daily or choosing a vegan diet are two of those good habits. Did you know that someone could choose habits like those and STILL NOT be healthy? On the other hand, someone can implement habits like working out and choosing a vegan lifestyle along with other good habits that are catered to the mind and body and be considered healthy even though his or her external appearance may not look the way you think it should look.

The word "health" is what I call a buzzword. It's one of those words that when you hear it, you automatically think of a generic body or mind functioning correctly. The reality is that the true definition of health isn't black and white. It is relative and specific to each person. There are certain habits that science has proven that contribute to health like appropriately hydrating the body, providing the body with the appropriate amount of activity, acquiring an appropriate amount of sleep, and consuming a balanced diet of fruits, vegetables, fats, and proteins. These are habits that can be beneficial to most people, and most times, this is where I advise my patients and clients to start. Acquiring health is a process. It's not something that happens overnight or by the push of a button. However, if you practice good habits consistently, you will experience good results over the course of your health journey.

It's important to note that in this instance, the journey means more than the destination. For example, if you wish to lose 50 pounds, and you accomplish your goal in a period of two weeks, though you most certainly would have accomplished your goal, the way in which it was done would have been very unhealthy and not done in a sustainable manner. When you define health for yourself, the key to success is to employ winning strategies that are sustainable and create small goals that you can modify at different points along the journey. The summation of these smaller goals in smaller increments eventually will result in a large primary goal. Instead of losing 50 pounds in two weeks, it is now a stepwise succession of losing 5 pounds the first week, maybe 7 pounds the second week, maybe another 5 pounds the third week, a whopping 8 pounds the fourth week, maybe 6 pounds the next week, and so on. If you utilized this strategy, you would not only lose the weight working towards your goal but also you are creating new habits in your new health spectrum. This way is much more effective than to take two steps forward and then five steps back and fall back into bad habits due to inadequate training, discipline, and what I call "fire hydrant goal stepping." You can't accomplish even the simplest task (i.e. drinking) effectively if it's coming out of a fire hydrant at full blast. You must take steps to slow down the flow of water to a level that is sustainable even when it comes to drinking water.

The bottom line in achieving true health is being consistent and complete in mind, body, and spirit. Being complete doesn't mean you won't experience periods of illness that are either acute (short-term) or chronic (long-term). Complete, in this instance, simply means having all of the necessary or appropriate parts or progressing to the greatest extent or the highest degree. Becoming complete in health is a continuous journey that you'll travel for the rest of your life. As previously discussed, mind and body health are directly correlated with one another. While the *appearance* of health is what most people desire, what's most important is the *expression* of health from the inside out. This expression of health is apparent in how quickly your body is able to adapt to changes in its environment. I always say if the inside functions, the outside will follow. This principle means the majority of your efforts should be focused on attaining health internally for the purpose of the cohesive and synergistic functioning of all your body systems.

God created us uniquely different from the hair on our head to the soles of our feet and even down to the cells and DNA in our body. As a result, *health* looks different on everyone. Knowing YOUR specific definition of health is a part of knowing YOU on a deeper connection beyond your external appearance and down to the internal workings of your very life. Let's help you define what "health" looks like for you.

MY GLOW UP

Give yourself grace. Health is a journey, not a destination. Since you have to be on this journey for the rest of your days, you might as well make it enjoyable, right? Know the difference in you for what "looks like" health and what actually is health. Your body is magnificently made and able to withstand A LOT of brutality. Just because it can doesn't mean it should. Don't be afraid to take control of your health so that you can thrive. After all, you're the only one who can.

CHAPTER

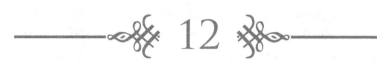

Your Mother Was Right! A Reasonable Bedtime Is Good For You

I remember a time when I was a little younger, in my twenties, in college, and living "the life." I recall having the ability to stay up to the wee hours of the morning only to catch a 2-hour nap and wake up to push through a full day of classes. Ironically, I was a pharmacy major then. I didn't consume any stimulants to keep me awake. I simply could survive off very little sleep or so I thought. I soon realized that I performed better in my classes when I was well-rested. Try taking an Organic Chemistry exam with 2 hours of sleep. At some point, it either becomes really funny and/or really scary. Neither option is good. As I matured years later, I perfected the idea of working smarter, not harder. I learned that I could accomplish more in less time with the appropriate amount of sleep. I could have used this epiphany in college, but I suppose it's better late than never that I learned this lesson.

It is important for you not only to understand sleep but also recognize the important role it plays in the sustainability of life. In fact, most people view sleep as an option as opposed to a necessity. I'm going to provide for you a brief overview or crash course of what sleep is in the body and why we need so much of it. I have this saying, "Never underestimate a good night's sleep." Sleep is essential for a number of reasons. First, it allows the body to rest and restore its energy levels. While it is seemingly a passive activity, the body actually is very active as it works diligently to repair and reproduce itself while storing energy for the next day. Remember when your mom would send you to bed if you didn't feel well? Better than that, what do you do most of the time you are feeling ill and trying to recover from an illness? You SLEEP! The same benefits exist when combating stress and attempting to solve complex problems. Why do you think people use the phrase, "Why don't you sleep on it and get back with me" when it comes to making major decisions? That's because sleep gives the brain a reboot or reset to clear the clutter and encourages mental clarity in making decisions and solving problems.

In an effort not to get too technical, Webster's Dictionary defines sleep as the natural, easily reversible periodic state of many living things that is marked by the absence of wakefulness and by the loss of consciousness of one's surroundings; it is accompanied by a typical body posture such as lying down with the eyes closed, the occurrence of dreaming, and changes in brain activity and physiologic functioning. It is made up of cycles of non-REM sleep and REM sleep and is usually considered essential to the restoration and recovery of vital bodily and mental functions. In short, sleep is a naturally occurring state characterized by reduced or absent consciousness, relatively suspended sensory activity, and inactivity of nearly all voluntary muscles. It's distinguished from wakefulness by a decreased ability to respond to stimuli (i.e. someone calls your name, and you don't respond.)

According to The Cleveland Clinic (2012) and The National Institute of Health (2016), sleep consists of two distinct states known as NREM (Non rapid eye movement) and REM (rapid eye movement) sleep. NREM sleep is subdivided into four stages: stage 1, stage 2, stage 3, and stage 4. Stages 3 and 4 collectively are referred to as slow-wave sleep or deep asleep. REM sleep may be subdivided into two stages:

phasic and tonic. Here is a crash course on what happens during each phase. Understanding sleep in detail often can provide clues as to why you may have trouble sleeping. More importantly, this information may hold the key to getting your sleep back to 6-8 hours each night.

The period of NREM sleep is made up of stages 1 through 4. Each stage can last from 5 to 15 minutes with stages 2 and 3 repeating backwards as the longer periods of stage 3 happen in the first half of the night before the body attains REM sleep.

STAGE 1

Have you ever heard the term "cat nap" or dozed off for a few minutes hoping it would energize you only to find that you feel just as tired and feel as if you haven't slept at all? Maybe you've even fallen asleep and didn't even realize it? Man, I remember being in professional school and trying to recover from midterms. We were on the quarter system, and our midterms were like one man playing against a whole team... ridiculous. We would take on average, 9-12 exams in a five day period. Recovering from this schedule was something that I both needed and wanted due to the fact that I was managing rigorous exam and study schedules. One particular day, I was dozing off in class, (or as I say... bobbing for apples) and I just could not find that spark in me to perk up and remain awake. The more I dozed, the sleepier I became. I tried going for a walk around the building and outside, and nothing helped. I was simply digging myself deeper and deeper into a hole. Stage one of REM is activated when you are dozing or nodding off. This is clearly where I was. During this stage, alpha and theta waves are active, and eye movements slow down. This is also the lightest stage of sleep in which you are aroused easily. This stage may last for 5 to 10 minutes, and often, people view it as a transition from wakefulness and sleep.

STAGE 2

Stage 2 is a period of light sleep. It offers the added benefit of a burst of energy. Waking after this stage of sleep is referred to as power naps. My daughter has these ALL of the time to the point that we have to use strategies with her sleep schedule. Sometimes, I try my hand at laying her down when she falls asleep in my arms. She is a one-year-old, so as you can imagine, if she's not past stage two, she has a very high likelihood of waking up despite my ninja moves when I try to lay her down. Are there any more moms out there who can relate to my experience? Stage two of NREM demonstrates sleep spindles with intermittent peaks and valleys of spontaneous, rapid, rhythmic brain activity that leaves you less aware of your surroundings. As a result, the body temperature decreases, and the heart rate and breathing slow and become more regular. This stage of sleep lasts for approximately 20-60 minutes as the body prepares to enter deep sleep. According to the American Sleep Foundation, people spend approximately 50% of their total sleep in this stage. (Suni, 2020)

STAGES 3 AND 4

Stages 3 and 4 are deep sleep stages. Stage 4 is more intense than stage 3. Fireworks occur during stages 3 and 4 of the NREM process. The body repairs and regenerates tissues, builds bone and muscle, and appears to strengthen the immune system. During deep sleep, your blood pressure and breathing rate decrease, and your muscles relax which makes it harder for you to be awakened. You are less responsive to external stimuli, and your body moves into a more restorative state in stage 4 of the NREM process. This stage of sleep lasts approximately 20-40 minutes. According to the Cleveland Clinic (TCC, 2012), as you get older, you get less NREM sleep. People under the age of 30 have about two hours of restorative sleep every night while those over the age of 65 might get only 30 minutes.

REM SLEEP

REM sleep is also referred to as a paradoxical sleep. During REM sleep, the brain becomes more active, the eyes move rapidly in different directions, the heart rate and blood pressure increase, and breathing becomes faster, more irregular, and shallower than normal resting inhalations. The muscles are more relaxed. The body becomes immobilized, and the brain's activity increases which leads to vivid dreaming. You generally enter REM sleep 90 minutes after falling asleep initially, and each stage lasts up to an hour for an average of five to six cycles each night. The American Sleep Foundation found that 20-25% of the total sleep people experience occurs in this stage (Suni 2020). It is important to note that age plays a role in how long you remain in each stage of sleep. For instance, infants will spend more time in REM sleep while adults will spend more time in NREM sleep.

Now that you understand the physiology of sleep, let's explore what it really is. You might find that you live a life that is always busy. Between working, taking care of the family, running errands, and finding time to relax and decompress (if there is any), oftentimes, sleep gets what's left over, which isn't a lot. Most people tend to think of sleep in terms of how rested they feel each day. However, the truth about sleep is that it's essential for bodily functions. From the outside, it may seem as though the brain and body shut down while you're sleeping, but as you just learned, it is both restorative and essential for cell building. The reality is well-rested people operate at a different level than people operating on as little as 1 to 2 fewer hours of sleep.

Loss of sleep impairs brain function and affects your higher levels of reasoning, problem solving, and attention to detail. These deficits make you less productive. It also influences your mood and increases your risk of depression. Aside from the brain, it affects every tissue and system in the body including growth and stress hormones, the immune system, appetite, breathing, blood pressure and cardiovascular health. Research has shown that a lack of sleep increases the risk for obesity, heart disease, and infections which also coincides with some of the leading causes of death. What exactly happens when we sleep? Throughout the night, your heart rate, breathing rate, and blood pressure rise and fall. This process is integral to cardiovascular health. Your body releases hormones during sleep that help repair cells and control the body's use of energy which subsequently has a large effect on the regulation of body weight. If getting sleep does ALL of that, can you imagine what not getting sleep does to your body? There is a reason why sleep deprivation is used as a form of torture. Some effects of sleep deprivation are listed below.

Effects of Sleep Deprivation

- Aching muscles
- Confusion, memory lapses or loss
- Depression
- Hallucinations
- Hand tremors
- Headaches
- Periorbital (eye) puffiness
- Increased blood pressure
- Increased stress hormone levels
- Increased risk of diabetes
- Irritability
- Nystagmus (involuntary eye movements up/down, side to side, or circular)
- Obesity
- Temper tantrums in children
- Yawning

- Symptoms similar to ADHD & psychosis
- Impaired immune system
- Risk of heart disease
- Growth suppression
- Decreased reaction time and accuracy

How many effects of sleep deprivation have you experienced? I would assume one too many. So, you may be asking, what is a good night sleep? Though it varies by age, a good night of sleep for adults consists of four to five sleep cycles. Figure 3-2b outlines the average amount of sleep needed per age group.

Figure 3-2. (CDC, 2017)

Age	Recommended amount of sleep per day
Newborn	Up to 18 hours
1–12 months	14–18 hours
1–3 years	12–15 hours
3–5 years	11–13 hours
5–12 years	9–11 hours
Adolescents	9–10 hours
Adults, including elderly	7–8 hours
Pregnant women	8(+) hours

Now, let's be honest. Sleep disruptions are real and can be plentiful. Stimulants such as caffeine or certain medications can limit sleep. Distractions such as electronics, the light from TVs, cell phones, tablets and e-readers also impair sleep. As you get older, illness, medications, and sleep disorders also can limit the amount of sleep that people get each night. As many as 70 million Americans of all ages suffer from chronic sleep problems with the two most common sleep disorders being insomnia and sleep apnea. Studies also have shown that a lack of sleep may increase the risk of Alzheimer's disease, osteoporosis, and cancer. Yes, most of us have experienced occasional insomnia at some point in time. Chronic insomnia, however, is defined as having trouble falling or staying asleep and lasting at least three nights per week for more than a month. It can trigger serious daytime problems such as exhaustion, irritability, and difficulty concentrating. Sometimes, relaxation exercises and deep breathing techniques are helpful in aiding those individuals with insomnia.

Sleep apnea is characterized by a loud, uneven snore in which breathing repeatedly stops or becomes shallow. Undiagnosed sleep apnea can be very dangerous because when very little air is exchanged for 10 seconds or more at a time, the oxygen decreases causing the body's fight-or-flight response to activate. Subsequently, your blood pressure spikes, your heart rate fluctuates, and the brain wakes you up partially to start your breathing again. This cycle creates a stress response, and when it is repeated, this response can leave you feeling tired and moody. Common therapies include sleeping on your side, exercising, or losing weight to reduce symptoms for mild cases. For more severe cases, a doctor may prescribe a patient a CPAP machine to pump air into the patient's throat to keep the airway open during sleeping. A bite plate that moves the lower jaw forward is also an option your doctor may prescribe. In severe cases, a patient may need surgery to address the sleep disorder. If you snore chronically and find that you wake up choking or gasping for air, you may need to be evaluated by your doctor who may order a sleep study for you to obtain an accurate picture of your sleep condition.

Below are some tips from the National Institute of Health for getting better quality sleep. (NIH, 2016)

GETTING QUALITY SLEEP

- Go to bed the same time each night and get up the same time each morning.
- Sleep in a dark, quiet, comfortable environment.

- Exercise daily (but not right before bedtime).
- Limit the use of electronics before bed (to include television).
- Relax before bedtime. A warm bath or reading might help.
- Avoid alcohol and stimulants such as caffeine late in the day.
- Avoid nicotine.
- Consult a health care professional if you have ongoing sleep problems.
- Meditation

My GLOW Up

Don't be a martyr for dirt and air. What I mean by that is don't sacrifice sleep for things that don't matter. Like breathing, sleep is fundamental. Don't allow anyone to convince you otherwise. Take time in your schedule to rest. Make it as essential as the food you eat or the money you make. Everything you have read builds upon itself. Effectively managing your stress greatly impacts the quality of sleep you will have. Make a promise to yourself to decompress at the end of the day so you can rest and reset to prepare adequately for the day ahead. Each day comes with it's own set of challenges, but if you prepare yourself well, you will be in a better position to conquer those challenges adequately instead of allowing the challenges to conquer you.

CHAPTER

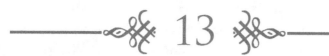

13

EAT, PRAY, BREATHE, LOVE... YOU ARE WHAT YOU EAT!

I remember talking amongst a group of friends a few years ago and laughing about the things our parents used to say to us that we now know were not only for our own good but also have migrated into our speech when we speak to our children or others we've encountered as adults. One of the most common phrases that has transcended culture and time is, "You are what you eat." Do you remember someone in authority saying that to you as a child? Most times, it came on the heels of not eating something that was healthy and undesired at the time.

The fact is our parents and parental figures were spot on! It wasn't just a trick to get you to finish your beets or brussel sprouts. Our bodies are literally composed of the food we eat. I would like to take it a step further and incorporate the childhood tale of "The Three Little Pigs." One pig built his house with straw. Another pig built his house with sticks, and the third pig built his house with bricks. We all know that the moral of the story is to use the proper materials to build your "house" to avoid the big bad wolf attempting to "huff and puff and blow your house down." The way in which you eat and the quality of foods you eat are analogous to the materials the little pigs used to build their respective homes.

When we eat a lot of processed material that the industry labels as "food", we find ourselves in the shoes of the little piggies that built their homes out of straw and sticks. However, when we are more diligent and educated regarding our food choices and choose organic and whole foods over non-organic and those foods with GMO, we are more like the little piggy who built his home out of bricks. The ability of the wolf, or sickness, disease, stress, etc., in our case, to affect our home and blow it down is related directly to the materials we use to build our homes. Your body is your first home. It existed long before you lived with your parents and moved out of their house and into your own home. When we are being formed in our mother's womb, the materials that her body uses to develop us are created from the food she consumes. Likewise, once we are born, we grow and develop based upon the nutrition we receive via the food we consume. It doesn't stop there. Did you know that different parts of your body replace themselves periodically while others remain with us from birth to death? Below is a chart of cell replacement of different organs and systems in the body.

Table. 3-3a Chart of Cell Replacement (Opfer, 2020)

Area of the Body	Time and/or Rate of Cell Replacement
Sperm cells	3 days
Colon cells	4 days
Red Blood cells	Every 4 months at an average rate of 100 million cells replacing the dying ones daily
Epidermis (Outer layer of skin)	Every 2-4 weeks

Gut epithelium (think lining of the stomach and intestines)	Every 2-9 days due to the constant exposure to digestive acids
Fingernails	Every 6 months
Scalp hair	Every 2-7 years. New ones fall out every day.
Bone	Every 10 years
Skeletal Muscle	Every 15 years
Fat cells	Every 25 years; Gaining and losing weight only affects the size of the cells and not so much the quantity.

There are a few items that stick around from birth to death which include half of the heart, the neurons in the brain (you are born with what you'll have), and the lens of the eye. Knowing that all of these items are replaced over the days, weeks, months, and years, the new cells have to be constructed from something, and that something is what we consume on a daily basis, food. Hence, **YOU ARE WHAT YOU EAT!** Told you they were right!

WHAT do you eat? Well, first, it's important to distinguish between diet and nutrition. Merriam Webster defines diet as either a food or drink regularly provided or consumed; the kind and amount of food prescribed for a person or animal for a special reason; or a regimen of eating and drinking sparingly so as to reduce one's weight. Nutrition, on the other hand, is defined as the process of nourishment or more simply the sum of the processes by which an animal or plant takes in and utilizes food substances. To simplify this a little more, I'd say that diet is what we consume, and nutrition is how we assimilate what we consume. Perhaps, if you think about it this way, diet is whatever you eat and is not specific to a name or trend. Your diet is simply what you chomp and swallow. Nutrition is the impact of how our body utilizes what we eat in terms of energy, building materials, etc. When we discuss diet in this text, we will refer to the regular consumption of food or drink. I will specify any other diets by name. Additionally, when it comes to diet, you must know that all food isn't created equally.

It is important to understand that the food/diet we consume now is NOT the food of our ancestors. They lived in a different time. Some might say they lived in a better time in some aspects. During our grandparents and great grandparents' childhood, organic food didn't have to be labeled because everything was organic! There was minimal processing of food which preserved its nutrients. Food was also more farm-to-table. Mass production of food occurred on a small scale, and companies utilized more human and ethical standards in their food production than they use currently. Gardens were plentiful, and the soil wasn't as depleted. The crops that grew were robust and filled with nutrients and minerals that came from living off the land. Farming and agriculture were plentiful unlike today. Now, our food and agricultural industries have moved backward in terms of standards. With this current new wave of health awareness, many people desire to go back to those days of their ancestors or at least incorporate aspects of those healthier practices within their current lifestyle.

Now, if food is our "straw, sticks, or brick," can you assess which material you are using the most to compose your house/body? There are numerous ways to approach nutrition and the diet that's best for you. I'm not talking about fad diets or trends but the foods your body chooses to eat. Note, I emphasized the food that your body chooses and not the foods that you choose. The reality of it is that our body knows EXACTLY what it needs, but our mind overcomplicates it. The media confuses us; the trends influence us; our family/friends don't understand us, and in the end, instead of listening to our body, we end up eating the wrong thing at the wrong time and pay the consequences later…cue fatigue, weakness, bloating, allergic reaction, unwanted weight gain, etc. Why go through all of this when you could listen to your body and feel energized and whole from the beginning?

As I've worked with my patients over the years, what I've learned is education is the missing and key component. One day, it dawned on me that people don't know what they don't know. If one doesn't know how to interpret the language of his/her own body effectively, how can he or she decipher possibly what his or her body needs at any given moment. The goal here is to help you foster a deeper relationship with your body to interpret appropriately the signals that will help you and your body function at its highest potential.

When you learn to listen to your body, you are better able to shut out the outside chatter of others or yourself for that matter. The way we are designed, and the way we eat are unique to each of us. Perhaps one of my favorite theories is bio-individuality, a concept coined by Dr. Roger Williams in his 1956 book titled *Biochemical Individuality*. In this text, he asserted that individuality permeates each part of the human body to include anatomy, metabolism, bodily fluid composition, cell structure, and even nutrition requirements. Largely ignored by mainstream medicine, this concept is adapted by a field of more independent thinkers in the worlds of health, nutrition, wellness, alternative medicine, etc.

Not only does this group understand some of his theories, but also this group often integrates them into their own lifestyles and practices. Most fad diets are regimented and mandate that everyone who enlists in them generally eats the same things. This is not a very individualized approach. We are way too individualized or unique to eat the same. Take a moment to think about the diverse people around you (family, friends, colleagues, etc.). Do you find that everyone's diet is exactly the same? Think about it. Women eat differently than men. We eat differently according to our age whether we are children, teenagers, young adults, middle aged adults, elderly, etc. Our differences vary with heritage, culture, and environment. Bio-individuality consists of a number of different options with regard to our bodies and food to include gender, ancestry, blood type, and metabolism. These are not the only aspects of bio-individuality that exist but certainly some of the most common.

When conversing with my patients and clients, many times women will complain that they have to cook two different meals or at the very least cook for two different tastes every night. They say things like, "I'm trying to transition to be a pescatarian, but my husband refuses to stop eating beef and chicken." They may say, "I'd love to try to go vegan to lose this weight, and all of my friends are doing it, but my husband refuses to let go of meat from his diet." (We'll unpack this last quote later on in the chapter.) The truth of the matter is that women, in large part, migrate easily to salads and light meals while men tend to desire heavier substances to include high protein meats and complex carbohydrates like potatoes and rice. Why is this? If you think back to our ancestors and their roles, the men always have been the heavy lifters and the workers outside of the home. Oftentimes, the men's work included manual labor which required increased calories to meet the demands of the body. Women, on the other hand, remained home and took care of the house which is NO SMALL FEAT; however, it required less heavy manual labor and energy needs. This is why a woman can have a salad for dinner 5 nights in a row and leave the table satiated and even full. However, a man can have a salad for dinner, but you may find him rummaging around the kitchen for a snack or small meal in the hours thereafter. It's because our diets are just as unique as we are. Now, does this apply to every man and every woman? Of course, this principle cannot be applied universally. Both men and women can run from one end of the spectrum to the other. It all depends on his/her lifestyle, caloric needs, and demands of the body for optimal function.

Table. 3-3b

Bio-Individuality – Ancestry (Rosenthal, 2006)

Geographical Region	Diet indigenous to that region
Japanese	Diet of rice, sea vegetables, and fish
India	Diet of basmati rice, cooked beans, and curry
Scandinavia	Ease of digesting dairy due to daily intake
Africa	Diet of beans, grains, animal protein, sweet potatoes, and green vegetables; difficulty digesting dairy due to limited access to dairy and trouble storing it in the region

BIO-INDIVIDUALITY – BLOOD TYPES (ROSENTHAL, 2006)

★The blood types are A, B, AB, & O. Most people may be unaware of their blood type, but research has shown that each blood type has developed specific strengths and limitations which significantly influence your health.

O – Tend to feel energized by eating meat and consuming high-protein foods; migrate towards eating lots of meat, vegetables, fish, and fruit but limit grains, beans, and legumes. To lose weight, seafood, kelp, red meat, broccoli, spinach, and olive oil are best; wheat, corn, and dairy are to be avoided.

A – choose fruit, vegetables, tofu, seafood, turkey, and whole grains but avoid meat. For weight loss, seafood, vegetables, pineapple, olive oil, and soy are best; dairy, wheat, corn, and kidney beans should be avoided

B – Tend to be better able to digest dairy; diverse diet including meat, fruit, dairy, seafood, and grains. To lose weight, type B individuals should choose green vegetables, eggs, liver, and licorice tea but avoid chicken, corn, peanuts, and wheat.

AB – Should eat dairy, tofu, lamb, fish, grains, fruit, and vegetables. For weight loss, tofu, seafood, green vegetables, and kelp are best but chicken, corn, buckwheat, and kidney beans should be avoided.

BIO-INDIVIDUALITY – METABOLISM

Have you ever met someone who was of a smaller stature but could eat more than your average amount of food? A common comment made to those individuals or by those individuals reflects the perception of a "high" metabolism. Some even comment about a high metabolism not knowing what it really means. They simply are able to notice the physical results of the person's eating practices. Metabolism, which is how you convert food into energy, varies by any number of factors including age, genetics, stress, etc. There are three general types of metabolic activity: fast burners, slow burners, and those who fall somewhere in between. Your fast burners are your protein types who tend to crave fatty, salty foods, are seemingly hungry ALL of the time, and don't function well on high carbohydrate or vegetarian-type diets because they burn through the fuel source too quickly. The slow burners are carbohydrate types who generally have weak appetites, LOVE sweets, and have subsequent weight control issues. These two exist on opposite ends of the spectrum where the high intake of carbohydrates speeds up their metabolism of the latter while the high intake of protein for fast burners tends to slow down their metabolism. Those who fall somewhere in between these groups have the best of both worlds with average appetites and moderate cravings of sweet, starchy, and salty foods.

What makes the individuality continue are the variables that can cause your metabolic rate and sensitivity to change. You can have shifts based on age, stress levels, nutrient deficiencies, hormonal changes and imbalances, or diet and lifestyle changes. Learning which one you are is as simple as a questionnaire or a medical test, but how do you keep up with the changes? That part is simple. You pay attention.

You remember that you are what you eat. You remember that you came from a unique ancestry of people who developed a system of eating based upon the environment in which they lived. Lastly, you remember that there is only one you, AND you are only given one body. While science and technology have made advances in medicine that allow for replacing parts and working wonders, when it all boils down to it, we are only given one body in this life. Like a car, we must make sure we are checking under the hood, paying attention to warning lights, getting tune ups and oil changes, and even getting detailed frequently to bring out that natural luster and shine that existed from the beginning. Pay attention to what you are eating. While this chapter focuses on the natural process of assimilating food and nutrients into the body, the book encompasses a blueprint of how to keep a new car new or restore a classic car back to its original condition before it experiences bumps and bruises, accidents, and failures.

There are many diets and fads that run across the television screen, scroll across social media, and entice people to decrease to their trimmest size so they can represent the stereotypical image of beauty. The foods you eat are meant to nourish your body so that it can replenish what is lost and replace what it needs. Knowing that you are what you eat, in the literal sense, should be enough to modify or at the very least cause you to be mindful of what you are putting in your body. If someone had a rare, hand-built Rolls Royce, you would hope that person would not put 87 octane gas in that classic car. Why? That type of car wasn't designed to handle that inferior quality of gas. The same thing applies to our bodies. Don't give it junk and then expect it to run like the best car in the world. In no way does that mean forgo ALL things deemed "not so healthy" and eat twigs and berries all of your life. What it does mean is that everything is acceptable in moderation. If you like french fries, please have them! Just don't eat them every other day. If you like steak, please have it. Just don't pair it with only potatoes and eat it 5 times a week. The key is that you need variety no matter your metabolic type and no matter the diet trends, etc. When we eat what we love, we tend to enjoy life just a little bit more. Fall in love with food again and allow it to contribute to your glow.

My GLOW Up

There is a lot that goes into eating. Can you just eat anything? Yes. Should you just eat anything? No. Should you enjoy eating? YES!! Eating should be joyous, so in your choices, remember to nourish your body and your soul. Don't forget that you are unique. The way your body assimilates food can be very different from that of a relative, stranger, or friend. Get to know you on a physical level and find the vibe that makes you thrive. When you find that vibe, your targets and goals will become easier to achieve, and life will become more enjoyable because you'll look good and feel good.

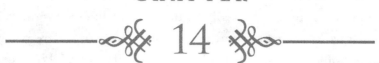

EXERCISE VS. FITNESS...
ARE THEY THE SAME?

Have you ever been in the gym or in the store, and you start sizing people up trying to estimate their level of fitness and judging them within that small increment of time? There was a time in my life when I did that. I'd find myself trying to do what they did. Even though I may have had more formal education at the time, it's just something about wanting to be in a certain place physically and the long journey it often takes to get there. I loved being in the gym and trying to out-lift or out-rep the one next to you. The crazy part is you do this when you have no knowledge of the person's journey, history, genetics, etc. You just know that the person may exhibit some of the physical attributes you desire. I quickly returned back to my goals and my journey, but this tends to happen to everyone at some point in his or her health and fitness path. Perhaps you've found yourself in this position before. You are slightly distracted by the success of others, and in the moment, you choose to emulate and replicate the person's actions in hopes of acquiring the same result.

By now, I'm sure you've noticed that I like definitions. They create clarity. First, let's determine the difference between exercise and fitness.

Do these two words have the same meaning? Do we as a society place more emphasis or differentiate one from the other? Let's dive in, shall we? If we look at the definitions, *exercise* is the activity requiring physical effort, carried out to sustain or improve health and fitness while *fitness* is the condition of being physically fit and healthy. Exercise is the vehicle by which we become fit. There are a million and one different ways to exercise. Some are traditional like running, lifting weights, etc., and others are non-traditional like gardening or climbing stairs. Here's the thing. It's okay to combine the traditional with the non-traditional so that you can arrive in a place where you are fit and healthy.

For many people, the reasons they desire to be fit are rooted often in superficial desires when the real reason should be because their lives depend on it. If you happen to have lives attached to you like a spouse or children, their lives depend on it too. While there are many, we will discuss the most important physiological aspects of incorporating exercise into your lifestyle.

Now, let's take a quick look at what happens in the body when we exercise. First, exercise requires energy. Sugar is stored in the body from the food we eat in the form of glycogen. The body uses glucose to create the energy the muscles use to contract which induces movement. Another familiar energy source our body uses is called adenosine triphosphate or ATP. Due to the small stores of glucose and ATP in our body, it needs more blood to be pumped into the contracting or exercising muscles to deliver the necessary oxygen used in the cycle to create more ATP. If less oxygen than needed is delivered, lactic acid will form instead. Typically, the body's lymphatic system will flush the lactic acid from the tissues within 30 to 60 minutes after exercise. The muscles grow larger as a result of micro tears in the tissue, and as healing takes place, soreness is the common result that notifies us of the changes in our muscular tissue.

As you exercise, your lungs also have to rise to the challenge. Depending upon the type of exercise that we perform, the body may require as much as 15 times more oxygen than normal. To achieve or meet these high demands, your respiratory rate will increase which will result in faster and heavier breaths from the musculature surrounding the lungs. This measurement is called the VO2 max, and it is used to determine the fitness level of a person. One of your fundamental breathing muscles outside of the lungs is known as the diaphragm. Like any other muscle in the body, the diaphragm can tire from improper movement. When it tires, people experience "side stitch" which is the feeling many runners experience when the diaphragm and its ligaments spasm.

One of the systems that exercise benefits the most is the cardiovascular system. As we exercise, the heart beats faster. As the heart rate increases, this causes the vascular system to circulate more blood delivering more oxygen at a faster pace. The more you exercise, the more efficient the heart becomes at this process which affords you the opportunity to exercise harder and longer to get faster and stronger. Ultimately, making the heart stronger will lower the resting heart rate in those who are fit. Because the heart is stronger, it is able to beat more efficiently and pump out more blood per pump each minute.

Exercise also stimulates the growth of new vascular tissue, namely new blood vessels. These new vascular units lower blood pressure in those who are fit. The increased blood flow from the resulting vasculature also benefits the brain, causing our neurons to function more efficiently. These effects translate to you feeling more alert and more focused even after you have finished your exercise.

Exercising regularly has been linked to lower rates and protection from diseases such as Alzheimer's, Parkinson's, and strokes. Additionally, exercise triggers chemical messengers of the brain called neurotransmitters. The most common of which are endorphins. You may be familiar with endorphins because they are often associated with the runner's high. This chemical interacts with the receptors in your brain that reduce your pain perception. Another neurotransmitter that gives a boost when exercising is serotonin. Serotonin is known for its role in mood and depression. What's even better is as oxygen and blood are delivered to the brain during exercise, the hippocampus, the area of the brain involved in memory and higher learning, is able to create new brain cells. The bonus is that even if you stop your exercise regimen (as we have all done before) we get to keep the new brain cells.

Last but not least, our pituitary gland which is housed in the control center of the brain alerts these small sacs located right above the kidney known as the adrenal glands. These glands have a direct linkage to stress. They also release the growth hormone when the body is in search of fuel to burn during exercise. Once the glycogen stores have been utilized, the body seeks another source of energy from either fat or muscle. The growth hormones released by the pituitary gland protect the muscles from being the first responders. That way you avoid burning off what you worked so hard to build.

Our kidneys filter impurities from our blood. The level of exertion or activity determines the rate of filtration. After periods of intense exercise, the kidneys allow greater levels of protein to be filtered in the urine. This response triggers a cascade resulting in better water re-absorption. Producing less urine keeps the body hydrated. One of the most common stress hormones the adrenal gland produces is cortisol. Cortisol is a key component in mobilizing the body's energy stores into fuel. Another hormone, adrenaline, causes a significant increase in the heart rate so that it can deliver and distribute blood throughout the body effectively and quickly.

The skin is another area that readily shows evidence of an increase in circulation. As exertion increases, the body like any other machine produces heat and needs to cool down. The blood vessels in the skin dilate or expand to accommodate the increased blood flow which allows the heat to dissipate through the skin into the air. This process creates a cooling mechanism. Eccrine and apocrine glands, two types of sweat glands, produce perspiration in the forms of salt water and electrolytes with the other glands producing fluid of a similar content that includes more fat. Perspiration is a cooling mechanism that aids the body in temperature regulation during exercise. Exercise can stress the joints up to five or six times more than our body weight with the primary and most active joints being the ankles, knees, hips, elbows, and shoulders. While all of these are different joints in terms of function and movement, each joint has a combination of fluid, cushioned tissue at the ends called cartilage, and elastic tissue connections called ligaments and tendons that provide stability.

Now that we know how the body responds to exercise and what exactly happens inside the body with exercise, it's practical application is knowing how to exercise appropriately to achieve your goals. When you want to build muscle, using high intensity activities for short periods of time is ideal. If the focus is losing fat, then low intensity activity for a longer duration will cause the body to deplete its glycogen stores and begin to burn fat instead. This depletion is caused by a calorie deficit during which you burn more calories than you've consumed. One thing we can be sure of is that no matter the activity, the body's response to exercise is the same while the results may manifest differently depending on a number of variables. Below you'll find a list of standard traditional exercises. Below that is another list which will include non-traditional options for exercise and activity. Are you a person who hates exercise? Then, go for the non-traditional route. Grab some friends and make it a date. Move about the city and keep it interesting. Don't get me wrong, there's nothing wrong with being in the gym, but there is something refreshing about a change of scenery. Why do you think people go on vacations? The change of scenery can trigger the release of endorphins in the body which improve our mood and increase our energy. One thing to remember is that there is always a way to be active whether you like it or not.

TRADITIONAL FORMS OF EXERCISE

- Running
- Resistance circuit training
- Weightlifting

- Cycling
- Jumping rope
- Swimming
- Walking
- Power walking
- Core Strength Exercises

NON TRADITIONAL FORMS OF EXERCISE

HIIT - High Intensity Interval Training- You're probably most familiar with Shaun T. and Beach Body's "Insanity" workout, but runners have been using interval training for more than 100 years as they alternate between sprinting and jogging to improve their endurance. This workout uses short bursts of high intensity movements with periods of rest or lower intensity training. What constitutes a high enough intensity is a heart rate at 80% of its maximum rate for one to five minutes. An example of this that you can try at home is the 10x1 which involves 10 one-minute bursts of exercise with each followed by one minute of recovery. Benefits include improved cardio-respiratory health with subsequent improvements in the VO2 Max. Incorporating this type of training with strength training can lead to increased muscle gains and strength.

Rowing - Have you ever done a Crossfit workout? If so, then you're no stranger to this puppy. A rowing machine simulates you rowing as if you're a part of a crew team except you're a team of ONE. It uses resistance, core, and body weight to propel the body forward and backward as you use your legs, arms, back, and core. Rowing, when done properly, targets 85% of your body's muscles. An added bonus of rowing is that it offers high intensity with a significantly decreased risk of injury. Rowing involves concentric muscle movement which causes tension in the muscle as it shortens while traditional exercises like squats are eccentric movements that cause tension on the muscles as they lengthen.

Dance - Dancing is a great way to work out without working out. More popular types include cultural dances like the salsa or African dance, while other popular culture dances like Hip Hop incorporate total body movement for extended periods of time. If someone asks you to workout with him or her at the gym for 4 hours, you might think he or she is crazy. If someone asks you to come dancing at the Latin club or attend a neighborhood party for 4 hours, it sounds much less crazy and way more fun. In addition to improving the cardiovascular system with the endurance component, strength training is involved as you move your body weight in various positions and maybe even with a partner! This is the epitome of working smarter not harder.

Hiking- What's better than exploring nature? Exploring nature and getting some exercise is an even better idea. Pack the necessities including plenty of water, a first aid kit, perhaps a snack or two, and you're off. As a weight bearing activity, you automatically will strengthen bones and muscles. Additional benefits of hiking include getting the oh-so-elusive Vitamin D! Allow the sunlight to shine, and your body will soak it up and process it for strong bones and a stronger immune system to combat cancer, autoimmune conditions, and depression. Walking and climbing with your pack builds the cardiovascular and respiratory systems as well.

Water Sports – If you live near a lake, try canoeing and kayaking, which provide excellent upper body workouts. You can try a paddleboard for paddleboard yoga, which provides a total body workout with an emphasis on the core. Paddleboard yoga is a more intense form of yoga in which your core is challenged as you attempt to perform those oh-so-interesting yoga poses while trying NOT to fall into the water. Not a fan of large bodies of water? No problem! Start off in a swimming pool. It'll do the trick, and you don't have to worry about any random wildlife coming to do yoga with you.

Ice Sports – If you're in a colder climate or smack in the middle of winter, incorporate some winter sports that will work the total body and increase your heart health. Ice skating, skiing, snowboarding, and even sledding provide awesome total body workouts. Working the muscles of the arms, legs, back, and core, is fun and entertaining for all.

Gardening- Gardening is one of those things that when done right, serves your body right times two! Whether you're a botanical genius, or you're exploring growing your vegetables in this unknown climate, playing in the dirt has its benefits. Brace the core to protect the lower back. Gardening involves bending, pulling, lifting, squatting, etc. It has all the makings of a full body workout with a delicious and healthy dinner to follow.

House Chores-What? Sounds crazy right? Think about the last time you gave your home a good scrub down and what you felt like afterwards. Is it coming back to you now? Picking up around the house, folding and putting up laundry, washing dishes, cleaning the bathroom, cleaning the floors, etc. require bending, lifting, reaching, pushing, pulling, and lots of movement. If you have a baby, multiply that times 100 because before they learn to walk, you are your baby's legs. From the very beginning, when they are as small as 3-8 pounds (or even pre-birth as you carry them as they grow) until they grow bigger and learn to walk and run at 25+ pounds, you do a lot of lifting. Maybe you're one of those people who finds cleaning therapeutic. Whether that's the life you live or not, a little motivation is always great. What better motivation is there than making it double duty and saving you that trip to the gym. Next time you are washing dishes or doing the laundry or the floors, pay attention to your body and brace your core for the entire time or at least at regular intervals. The added stability provided to your spine and torso helps you to tighten all of the muscles around your abdomen, and there are quite a few of them. Activate the muscles in your legs as you glide across the floor. Perform calf raises while standing at the sink doing the dishes. Make every move intentional and let that serve as a substitute for a couple of gym days.

In the end, there is no one-size-fits all approach for diet or fitness no matter how hard you try. The secret is finding your special combination unique to you to which your body will respond so you can achieve the results you seek. It's really about knowing your body or getting to know it and finding what resonates most with both your body and your spirit. You have to like and preferably love your activity. Otherwise, the element of consistency goes out of the window. Consistency is key in maintaining an active regimen above anything else.

MY GLOW UP

Don't let fitness become a chore. Get creative and make it fun! Non-traditional fitness can be just as effective. Get outside, even if it's just for 30 minutes. Your body needs sunlight to make the Vitamin D that makes you strong. Accountability is everything, so find a partner, enlist your significant other, or make it a family affair. Set good examples now to translate to healthy kids later. Fitness is more about quality than quantity. Start small and set aside increments of time, 15 minutes here and 15 minutes there. Be consistent and don't over-exert yourself. Treasure the treasure you have and let's get this work!

PART 4

EMOTIONALLY: MAKE TIME TO P.L.A.Y.

EPILOGUE

EAT, PRAY, BREATHE, *LOVE & GLOW!* MAKE TIME TO P.L.A.Y

Remember when you were a little kid in school, and no matter how much work you did or how many tests you took, there was always time to play. We call that recess! I don't know about you, but there was something about being able to release it all and just have fun and enjoy being a kid. There were the monkey bars, the slides, and the swings, and whether you were the type to find a tree and read a book or to run wild on the grounds, recess was EVERYTHING, and you made time to play.

How often do we as adults make time to PLAY? I mean that in the literal sense. How often do you take the time to enjoy this thing called life? I used to do the opposite of play. I worked as a student in school for many years, I worked as an adult in between degrees and life. I worked and worked and worked until I made the conscious decision one day that I would NOT work myself into oblivion. Actually, my husband and I decided together to have a better life, to LIVE a better balanced life intentionally, and to breathe ON PURPOSE. LIVE on Purpose. Exist on Purpose. Rear our children on Purpose. PLAY ON PURPOSE in both the literal and figurative sense. Today, I challenge you to make time for P.L.A.Y. (Prioritize, Love, and Appreciate the beauty of yourself and

Yield to your destiny.) Perhaps the deeper question is why don't you play already? Let's break this down a bit, and while this won't be a chapter full of mind-blowing revelations, it hopefully will provide you with some insight, clarity, and thought-provoking truths. This chapter will both challenge you and require you to complete it.

PRIORITIZE YOURSELF

Due to the many hats we wear and the roles we play, placing ourselves in the priority spot comes either rarely or never. Prioritizing is important for everyone except you (insert side eye) but why is that? Why is it that you work so hard to care for and nurture everyone else, but you don't take time for yourself? Self-care is huge, and self-investment is the gift that keeps on giving. When was the last time you invested in yourself? Now, answer this, when was the last time you invested in someone other than yourself? Do you like your two answers? Somehow, in society and modern culture, the understanding has been that it's ok to self-sacrifice, self-sabotage, and to give of yourself to everyone but you. The reality of this culture is flawed and detrimental not only to the survival of the strong, but also it both undermines and sets us back 100 years to the time when we were nothing more than familial units. Don't get me wrong. My roles as a wife and mother are two of the most powerful, most challenging, and most rewarding roles I've ever worn, but there is so much more to women during this time. Now, we can be literally ANYTHING we want, and yes, we are still fighting for equality in a lot of ways, but the reality is that we can be doctors, lawyers, politicians, accountants, entrepreneurs, and even the President of the United States of America, and we ARE!

Some confuse prioritizing yourself to mean that you prioritize your career, and while that is not wrong, it just isn't completely accurate or healthy. Working your way up the corporate ladder, fighting discrimination, making your mark, and staking your claim are all very wonderful steps and deserve accomplishments and accolades. For many, you prioritized your career in order to get to the place where you are but failed to prioritize yourself in the process. You invested in a title but not in a person. Start prioritizing yourself today. Start making decisions that will bring you joy PERSONALLY. Maybe that looks like you having a girls night once a month or a spa day when you need it. It can be something as simple as an hour of quiet time before the house rises in the morning or perhaps a time in the evening that's just as special. Whatever it is, the idea is for it to bring you joy...real joy...TRUE Joy.

LOVE YOURSELF

When was the last time you looked in the mirror and said the words, "I love you" to the reflection peering back at you? If your answer isn't today, last night, or a day or so ago, it's been too long. The sad truth is that some of us will express more love to our spouse and children than we would ever express to ourselves. Why is that? It comes down to a fundamental truth. There is a great number of women who don't love themselves, and what's worse, they will deny it to the bitter end. Sometimes, it's easy to hide behind a lie because the truth just sounds too horrible and is too painful. I'm a firm believer that you can't love others consistently and effectively until you unapologetically love yourself FIRST. Love is defined as an intense feeling of deep affection or a great interest or pleasure in something or a person or thing that one loves. Though these definitions are all a bit different, they are all accurate.

Answer the following questions as if no one is listening or watching because they aren't. Do you feel a deep affection (gentle feeling of fondness or liking) towards yourself? Do you have a great interest in yourself? Are you someone whom you love? How do you demonstrate that love daily? If you answered "No" to any or all of these questions, I say to you, "Congratulations!" You've made the first step by being honest about where you are. I sometimes have my clients repeat mantras throughout the day and definitely every time they see their reflection in the mirror. Why do I require them to do this? Repetition is key. We are creatures of habit. If you don't already, I'd like for you to participate with me. Whenever you pass by a mirror, look at your reflection and say the words, "I LOVE YOU, I LOVE ME." The "I love you" represents you loving the image you see staring back at you. The "I love me" represents the soul and spirit you inhabit that pushes you to live the life you live. It's a sense of taking responsibility and taking ownership of everything you are and everything you are NOT while loving ALL of it.

The second part of repeating that mantra is that you say it aloud, and even if you're in a public space (whisper it quietly). You do this so your ears can hear what your mouth is saying. Understand that loving yourself allows you to see who you really are including the good, the bad, and the indifferent. It's the first step in working on the parts of you that need work and accepting and embracing the parts of you that are beautiful whether society says so or not. Love ALL of you as Christ loves you. You deserve it.

APPRECIATE YOUR BEAUTY

Beauty is YOUR name. Those words are reminiscent of a song years ago that I would belt out around the house. (Don't act like you haven't had your belting out moments too.) When you prioritize and love yourself, self-appreciation is next if you are not doing that step already. When you appreciate something, you show the reverence or the value you have in that said object or person. When we look at the word, "appreciate," what does it mean? Perhaps it's the educator in me, but I love word definitions...Clearly! Definitions help me to develop a deeper understanding, at times, of what a word means. Thus, appreciate means to recognize the full worth or be grateful for something; understand (a situation) fully or recognize the full implications of; or a rise in value or cost. That last definition is a sermon in itself, right? When you look at yourself, do you recognize the full worth of who you see? This is HUGE. If you don't, why don't you? Worth is a funny thing. What one person feels is junk is another person's treasure. Guess what? You should see the treasure in you. Are you grateful for the person you are? The wife/husband you've become? The mother/father you are?

Being grateful for the beauty you possess both inside and out is a testament of how your experiences have shaped you and molded your beauty year after year. I must admit that the last part of the definition is my absolute favorite. Have you appreciated your beauty to assess your rise in value? Beauty has little to do with what's on the outside and everything to do with what's on the inside. I know it sounds cliché but it's true. Appreciating your beauty is all about the qualities that make you valuable to yourself and those attached to you. External beauty is fleeting and can change in an instant. Appreciate every part of who you are from the crown of your head to the soles of your feet. Appreciate the asymmetry of your facial features and your boobs from the baby you had years ago. Appreciate your whole body, the excess belly fat, that mole that you've been contemplating removing, your hair that only behaves when it absolutely wants to, and your feet which might be due for a pedicure. Embrace and appreciate ALL of those qualities because they are YOU. Your beauty deserves to be appreciated, and no one will appreciate your beauty until you appreciate it **first**.

YIELD TO YOUR DESTINY

At the end of the day, a WELL YOU is a HAPPY YOU. A HAPPY YOU makes for a HAPPY FAMILY with HAPPY children and the dog too. The key to being well is not in chasing down each fad that approaches. It's all about developing your own G.L.O.W. Rx so that you can **G**row and **L**ive **O**ptimally **W**ell. Does becoming well require more than heading to the gym a few days a week? Yes. Fitness is only one component. While most people think of wellness in terms of exercise and fitness, it is an all-encompassing term used to umbrella a number of broad topics that culminate into a WELL person in ALL facets of life.

Being a Well YOU requires that you make certain decisions to create a space for YOU where you feel loved, whole, safe, and at peace.

Becoming a Well YOU requires creating space in what seems like the tightest schedule so that you can be uplifted by others, but more importantly, you can be loved by you. Becoming a Well YOU means releasing fear, worry, angst, doubt, and façades into the wind to show up every day as yourself and no one else unapologetically.

A Well YOU means you aren't afraid to find your GLOW for fear of what's there or what someone else might say. It simply means yielding to the destiny that is yours and belongs to no one else. Choose to conquer your fears and take the leaps necessary to walk out your journey step by step. Remember, it is all a process. There is beauty and growth in the process. The prescription is written, and you have everything you need. This is the place where you stand and embrace your BEAUTIFUL body with self-love, self-appreciation, and self-care as a priority. It's time to level up. This...is your G.L.O.W. Rx.

REFERENCES

5 Things You Should Know About Stress. (n.d.). Retrieved November 07, 2018, from https://www.nimh.nih.gov/health/publications/stress/index.shtml

American Psychological Association (2017). Stress in America: The State of Our Nation. Stress in AmericaTM Survey.

ASA Authors & Reviewers Sleep Physician at American Sleep Association Reviewers and Writers Board-certified sleep M.D. physicians. (n.d.). Stages of Sleep: The Sleep Cycle. Retrieved June 12, 2020, from https://www.sleepassociation.org/about-sleep/stages-of-sleep/

Avgerinos, J., About the Author Jennifer Carter Avgerinos Certified Instructor: Yoga Jen is a creative and passionate writer, & Jen is a creative and passionate writer. (2016, June 23). 6 Ways to Create a Sacred Space at Home. Retrieved November 07, 2018, from https://chopra.com/articles/6-ways-create-sacred-space-home

Brock, F. (2019, September 02). Get To Know Yourself: 29 Questions to Discover the Real You. Retrieved September 25, 2020, from https://www.prolificliving.com/get-to-know-yourself/

Dictionary by Merriam-Webster: America's most-trusted online dictionary. (n.d.). Retrieved November 07, 2018, from https://www.merriam-webster.com/

Donne, J.(1624). Meditation 17. *Devotions Upon Emergent Occasions.* https://www.poemhunter.com/poem/no-man-is-an-island/

Gaiam, & Inner IDEA. (n.d.). Meditation 101: Techniques, Benefits, and a Beginner's How-to. Retrieved November 07, 2018, from https://www.gaiam.com/blogs/discover/meditation-101-techniques-benefits-and-a-beginner-s-how-to

Grayson, H., Ph.D. (2019, April 25). Mind Body Medicine: How to Uncover the Hidden Mental-Emotional Roots of Illness. Retrieved November 07, 2018, from https://www.consciouslifestylemag.com/mind-body-connection-health/

International Stress Management Association (2017). How To Identify Stress. https://isma.org.uk/how-to-identify-stress

Kuruvilla, C. (2016, March 04). How To Create A Sacred Space In Your Home. Retrieved November 07, 2018, from https://www.huffpost.com/entry/how-to-create-a-sacred-space-in-your-home_n_56d-72b12e4b03260bf78e917

Mascarelli, A. (2015, February 06). 5 Solutions to Common Meditation Excuses + Fears. Retrieved November 07, 2018, from https://www.yogajournal.com/meditation/answers-common-meditation-excuses-fears-experience

Opfer, C. (2020, January 27). Does your body really replace itself every seven years? Retrieved June 10, 2020, from https://science.howstuffworks.com/life/cellular-microscopic/does-body-really-re-place-seven-years.htm

Rosenthal, J. (2006). *Integrative nutrition: The future of nutrition.* New York City: Institute for Integrative Nutrition.

Stress: Signs, Symptoms, Management & Prevention. (2015, February 05). Retrieved November 07, 2018, from https://my.clevelandclinic.org/health/articles/11874-stress

Suni, E, Vyas, N. (2020, Aug 14). Stages of Sleep. *The Sleep Foundation* https://www.sleepfoundation.org/articles/stages-of-sleep

Taylor, J. (1978). *The Bible.* Rutland: Printed by Fay & Davison.

2016, May 1. A Good Night's Sleep. The National Institutes of Health. https://www.nia.nih.gov/health/good-nights-sleep#good

The Cleveland Clinic (2012). Sleep Basics. https://my.clevelandclinic.org/health/articles/12148-sleep-basics

The Whole Cure Lifestyle Transformation Mind Module. (n.d.). Retrieved from http://www.jenniferweinbergmd.com/product/wholecure-lifestyle-mind/

Understanding Sleep Cycles. (n.d.). Retrieved June 12, 2020, from https://www.sleep.org/articles/what-happens-during-sleep/

Weinberg, J., About the Author Jennifer Weinberg Preventive and Lifestyle Medicine Physician and Author Dr. Jennifer Weinberg, & Weinberg, D. (2019, October 23). Mind-Body Connection: Understanding the Psycho-Emotional Roots of Disease. Retrieved November 07, 2018, from https://chopra.com/articles/mind-body-connection-understanding-the-psycho-emotional-roots-of-disease

Williamson, M. (2019, April 23). A RETURN TO LOVE: Reflections on the Principles of A Course in Miracles. Retrieved September 25, 2020, from https://marianne.com/a-return-to-love/

CONNECT WITH ME

J ust like that, you're well on your way to wellness! I've shared with you my four pillars of health to nurture and build every aspect of your life so that you can be free and whole. If you would like to obtain a greater understanding and garner more support and accountability, I have just the thing for you. Below, you'll find a few resources to help you get started and assist you along your journey.

Coaching and Consulting

If you are in need of direct support and guidance while crafting an Rx plan that is just for you, I've got you covered. Learn more about my services and programs on my website, **www.drnicolemccarty.com** and we'll get you together.

Corporate Wellness & Education

My corporate wellness programs are more than just ergonomics and the daily step count. Don't get me wrong, those are great, but I think we can all agree, especially after reading *GLOW Rx*, that wellness is so much more than that. Our program, "Wellness in the Jungle," incorporates professional development, leadership development, and health and wellness development to impact and create complete people who become complete employees. Productivity increases. Work culture increases. Morale increases. Revenue increases. It's a win all around. You can learn more about my programs at **www.drnicolemccarty.com.**

Consulting & Speaking

The application of knowledge is the key to success. A great passion of mine is sharing my knowledge with others. *Each one, reach one, teach one* is a motto by which I live. For more information on booking engagements and workshops, please visit, **www.drnicolemccarty.com/ connect**.

I'd love to connect with you online at any of the following social media platforms!

Facebook: https://www.facebook.com/DrNicoleMcCarty
Instagram: https://www.instagram.com/dr.nicolemccarty/
Twitter: https://www.twitter.com/DrNicoleMcCarty
LinkedIn: https://www.linkedin.com/in/
    dr-nicole-mccarty-80556062/
Website: www.drnicolemccarty.com
YouTube: Dr. Nicole McCarty

ABOUT THE AUTHOR

r. Nicole McCarty is by definition, a logic driven, "personal energy conservationist", a thinker, a lover of laughter, & lover of life. She is also a health enthusiast. As a sports chiropractor, yoga instructor, biomechanics and soft tissue specialist, and owner of The WELLYOU Bar, she is a collegiate professor at Life University, speaker, corporate wellness facilitator, health & wellness coach, and entrepreneur. She has experience in virtually every sector of the health and wellness industry which includes work as a hyperbaric oxygen specialist, a respiratory therapist (graduate of the incomparable Florida A&M University...Rattler Pride), a sports chiropractor, a yoga instructor, and also as trained birth doula (go figure). Perhaps more than anything, she is a wife, a mom, a managing caregiver for her grandparents, and a lover of God and people!

Dr. McCarty is passionate about all things related to health. Her desire is to create a space where people can start and continue the journey of becoming Well in addition to becoming the very BEST version of themselves in spite of busy schedules, fear, and a lack of knowledge. The WellYOU Bar is more than a fitness space or doctor's office for that matter. Consider it an oasis of well being where we believe in taking an integrative and holistic approach to health, nurturing the physical, mental, emotional, and spiritual part of you. It is a haven and community dedicated to self-care and restoration through education and demonstration. We accomplish this via a focus on health and wellness coaching/strategy services and on corporate wellness needs. The corporate wellness component caters to leadership and wellness development from the inside out in team environments for increased client retention.

As a bit of bonus insight, beyond a free spirit, Dr. McCarty is more of an introvert than an extrovert but LOVES, LOVES, LOVES what she does and how she's been able to help transform people's lives literally. What drives her is using her gifts to bless others, and for her, it simply doesn't get better than that. She finds purpose and great joy in knowing and living a life of freedom, health, wellness. Purpose is everything. Freedom is her mantra of sorts, so much so that she's got the ink to prove it. She knows and teaches the benefits of freedom. Her desire is for every individual to experience a glimpse of freedom to know that they too, can have that same level of it and then proceed to move heaven and earth to get there.

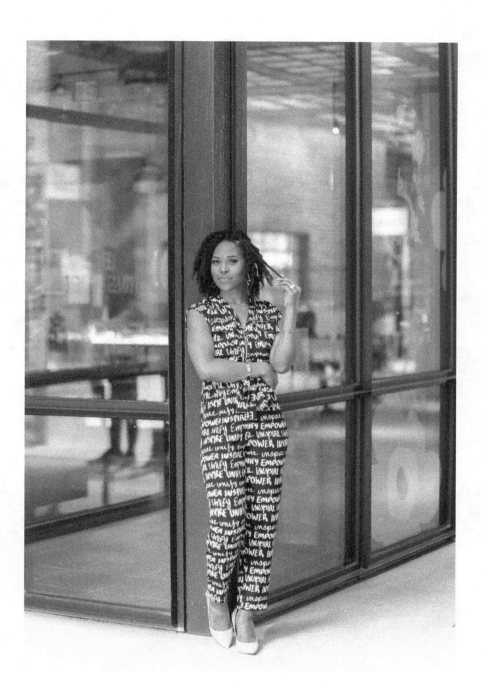

CPSIA information can be obtained
at www.ICGtesting.com
Printed in the USA
JSHW031519030221
11490JS00001B/41

9 781735 984506